WOMEN'S HEALTH AND FITNESS

THE NO NONSENSE LIBRARY

NO NONSENSE HEALTH GUIDES

Women's Health and Fitness
A Diet for Lifetime Health
A Guide to Exercise and Fitness Equipment
How to Tone and Trim Your Trouble Spots
Stretch for Health
Unstress Your Life
Calories, Carbohydrates and Sodium

NO NONSENSE FINANCIAL GUIDES

NO NONSENSE REAL ESTATE GUIDES

NO NONSENSE LEGAL GUIDES

NO NONSENSE CAREER GUIDES

NO NONSENSE SUCCESS GUIDES

NO NONSENSE COOKING GUIDES

NO NONSENSE WINE GUIDES

NO NONSENSE PARENTING GUIDES

NO NONSENSE HEALTH GUIDE®

WOMEN'S HEALTH AND FITNESS

A Take-Charge Plan for Lifetime Well-Being

By the Editors of
Prevention® Magazine

Longmeadow Press

Notice

This book is intended as a reference volume only, not as a medical manual or guide to self-treatment. It is not intended as a substitute for the medical advice of physicians. The reader should regularly consult a physician in general, and particularly for any symptoms. If you suspect that you have a medical problem, we urge you to seek competent medical help. Keep in mind that exercise and nutritional needs vary from person to person, depending on age, sex, health status and individual variations. The information here is intended to help you make informative decisions about your health, not as a substitute for any treatment that may have been prescribed by your doctor.

Women's Health and Fitness

Published April 1987 for Longmeadow Press, 201 High Ridge Road, Stamford, CT 06904.

Library of Congress Cataloging-in-Publication Data

Women's health and fitness.

(No-nonsense health guide)
1. Women—Health and hygiene. 2. Physical fitness for women.
3. Women—Medical care. I. Prevention (Emmaus, Pa.) II. Series. [DNLM:
1. Gynecology—popular works. 2. Health. 3. Physical Fitness—popular works. 4. Women—popular works.
WP 120 W8717]
RA778.W754 1987 613'.0424 87-4165
ISBN 0-681-40134-6 paperback

Special thanks to Catherine Cassidy for compiling and editing the information in this book.

Book design by Acey Lee and Lisa Gatti

Photographs by Carl Doney p. 24, top; T. L. Gettings pp. 24, bottom, 25, bottom; Ed Landrock p. 25, top.

No Nonsense Health Guide is a trademark controlled by Longmeadow Press.

2 4 6 8 10 9 7 5 3 paperback

Contents

Lessons in Women's Health Care

Women live longer than men. A typical female born in 1900 outlived a typical male by two years. And the lead is growing. Women born in 1980 can expect to live 7½ years longer than their male counterparts. No one is quite sure why. Researchers cite various theories, crediting different sets of genes, different combinations of hormones—and possibly different health habits.

One major difference seems to lie in the way women and men approach illness. Ironically, health surveys show that women report more acute illnesses and symptoms than men do. But women aren't necessarily less healthy than men. They do, however, seek medical help more often than men, which increases their chances of early diagnosis and treatment and may give them valuable information about their own health. The masculine stereotype, on the other hand, discourages many men from admitting to weakness or pain and seeking help of any kind.

Perhaps women have a more keenly developed skill of listening to their bodies, too. Menstruation and the physical and emotional changes that accompany it have a way of tuning a woman in to her internal environment early in life. So does the way reproductive organs are arranged. Tucked away in a dark, moist environment, for example, the vagina and the nearby urinary tract are host to all sorts of troublesome bacteria, viruses and fungi. So sooner or later, most women will have to deal with some degree of itching, inflammation or other unpleasantness related to sex or reproduction.

Sometimes symptoms call for medical help and sometimes they don't: The trick is to be able to tell the difference. And when a problem does call for medical attention, the better-informed consumer is apt to get better care. Until the women's rights movement of the 1960s and 1970s, many women felt that doctors didn't take their health concerns seriously and were all too likely to respond to their questions with a pat on the head and a "No need to worry" than with any substantial information. Worse, doctors seemed to hold a common belief that women often had psychosomatic illnesses. In fact, one study found that women were as much as 60 percent more likely to receive a prescription for a tranquilizer than men who saw a doctor for the same complaint. Critics contend, too, that women seem to be the victims of much unnecessary surgery. It is estimated that as many as 40 percent of all the hysterectomies performed are unnecessary. And five of the ten most common procedures with medical risk involve women's reproductive organs.

So a women's health movement has evolved in the wake of the women's rights movement. A little hypochondria, it seems, is healthier than denial—or a totally submissive attitude toward medical help. Women's rights activists—even doctors themselves—have encouraged women to learn more about menstrual problems, pregnancy, childbirth, birth control options, weight control, nutrition, stress reduction and other aspects of preventive health care. The goals are to minimize short-term problems and to prevent them from becoming long-term problems.

Weight control is one area where being better informed leads to better health. We now know that being thin *in itself* is not necessarily healthy, but *how* you slim down is crucial. Starving yourself down to a size 8 can do more harm than good, leaving you nutritionally deprived on the inside and still soft and flabby on the outside. Exercising your way into shape, on the other hand, builds muscle while it burns fat, leaving you slimmer yet still able to carry your own luggage or climb a flight of stairs without getting out of breath. In effect, a new, more appropriate definition of women's fitness shifts the emphasis from outward appearance to total health.

Women have developed healthier psychological attitudes, too. In its zeal to lead women everywhere to self-fulfillment, the women's movement initially left many women feeling cheated unless they had a brilliant career *and* ran a perfect household *and* raised perfect children *and* rotated their own tires (*and* pretended this balancing act was mere child's play). Now we're smarter. A second wave of feminism says, "Let's not be so hard on ourselves, or we'll lose that seven-year lead in longevity, to say nothing of our sanity." It's okay to devote your energies to motherhood and motherhood alone, if you wish. You don't have to be chairperson of the board. (You don't even have to *want* to be chairperson of the board.) It's even okay to ask a mechanic (male or female) to work on your car. Just so you have enough information to make the right choices.

That's what this book is all about: choosing better health. We hope this information will help you to choose a sound diet; to determine the right course of action if you have menstrual discomfort; to put together an exercise routine that will get you in shape gradually, without strain or injury; to point out not one but several ways to handle stress. In short, we hope this information will help you to establish a personal long-range health and fitness plan that takes into account the special needs that arise from being a woman.

C H A P T E R

O N E

Bridging the Nutritional Gender Gap

Studies show that men and women eat differently and that they have distinct nutritional needs.

Food preference surveys, for instance, show that men are nearly twice as likely as women to eat whatever they want, and what they want is a high-fat cut of red meat. That's one reason that, even in these health-conscious times, the typical man's diet is too high in fat and sometimes low in the vitamins and minerals found in fruits, vegetables and dairy products.

Women like meat, too, but they also want fruits and vegetables. Their food shopping and cooking skills make them likely to be more nutritionally aware than men, but they also have special dietary demands, particularly during pregnancy. And they're twice as likely as men to be watching their weight and thus possibly eating too few calories to supply all the nourishment they need, especially during their childbearing years.

The Recommended Dietary Allowances (RDAs) established by the Food and Nutrition Board of the National Research Council reflect most but not all of the differences in nutritional requirements between the sexes. At every age men require 10 to 30 percent more protein, vitamins A, E and B_6, thiamine, riboflavin, niacin and magnesium than women. They require the same amount of vitamins D, C and B_{12}, folate, calcium, phosphorus, zinc and iodine. They require only about half as much iron. (See the table on pages 4 and 5 for the recommended daily intake of essential vitamins and minerals for women.)

Women who are pregnant or breastfeeding an infant have the highest nutritional requirements. They need vitamins and minerals in amounts equal to or greater than those required by men. In some cases—with folate and calcium, for instance—their needs jump dramatically. Not meeting those needs can result in a low-birth-weight baby or seriously impair the mother's health.

Iron Requirements

Iron is one nutrient women need more of than men, according to the Food and Nutrition Board. Menstruating women require almost twice as much iron as men (18 milligrams compared to 10 milligrams), and pregnant women may need 30 to 60 milligrams of iron each day.

Nutritional surveys show that about 40 percent of women of childbearing age don't get enough iron, says Cecilia Davis, a registered dietitian who directs a nationwide dietitian's referral service, the Consulting Nutritionist Practice Group.

"Women absorb only about six milligrams of iron per 1,000 calories of food in a typical diet," she says. "They would need to eat about 3,000 calories a day to meet their iron RDA. Few eat that much, so many women need supplemental iron."

Teenage girls are even worse off, Davis contends. "I'd say 80 percent could be iron deficient. Some eat as few as 1,000 calories a day, and their food preferences are poor in iron."

Both adult men and women may sometimes become iron depleted during very strenuous athletic training, says Paul Zabetakis, M.D., a research physician at the Institute of Sportsmedicine and Athletic Trauma in New York. In superathletes, pounding exercise can actually break down red blood cells and lead to anemia (iron deficiency).

Dr. Zabetakis cautions that average runners as well as ultramarathon athletes may develop "pseudo-anemia." Blood tests will show lower-than-normal iron levels, but the larger volume of blood developed as a result of athletic activities means the oxygen-carrying capacity remains the same. The athletes will have no physical symptoms of anemia.

When most adult men (and women past menopause) develop iron deficiencies, though, it's usually not exercise or diet that's at fault, says Robert McGandy, M.D., a Tufts University professor of medicine and consulting physician for the Boston-based Human Nutrition Research Center on Aging. Internal bleeding—from ulcers, intestinal polyps, excessive aspirin or alcohol use and even hemorrhoids—is too often the cause. "In this case, it's important to be checked for blood loss and not to try to cure yourself with an iron supplement," Dr. McGandy says.

Mother's Helper: Folate

Sometimes what masquerades as an iron deficiency is actually a folate problem. One common nutritional problem in the United States is a low intake of this B vitamin. People just aren't eating enough folate-rich, dark green leafy vegetables, and women especially pay the consequences.

Anemia can occur when there is not enough folate in the body to produce red blood cells. Especially among older women, folate rather than iron may be the culprit in this problem. And folate deficiencies have been implicated in cervical dysplasia, a condition that can lead to cancer of the cervix. The vitamin has also been found to reverse dysplasia in some women.

Pregnant women need to double their folate intake from 400 to 800 micrograms, and those who are breastfeeding need 500 micrograms. "Folate is needed for the manufacture of all cells," Dr. McGandy says. That's why it's so important for fetal growth and growth of the newborn baby. In fact, both spina bifida, a birth defect in which the tissue around the spinal cord doesn't close properly, and cleft palate have been associated with low folate intake. In one study, women who had had one baby with spina bifida were much less likely to have a second baby with the same problem if they got adequate folate.

Special Needs for B_6

Vitamin B_6 has been associated with "women's problems" for some time now. It's been used to treat fluid retention and other symp-

(continued on page 6)

Recommended Dietary Allowances (per Day) for Women

Vitamins

	Age (yr.)	Weight (lb.)	Height	Protein (g.)	Vitamin A (I.U.)	Thiamine (mg.)	Riboflavin (mg.)	Niacin (mg.)	Vitamin B_6 (mg.)	Vitamin B_{12} (mcg.)	Folate (mcg.)	Vitamin C (mg.)	Vitamin D (I.U.)	Vitamin E (I.U.)
All Women	11-14	101	5′2″	46	4,000	1.1	1.3	15	1.8	3.0	400	50	400	12
	15-18	120	5′4″	46	4,000	1.1	1.3	14	2.0	3.0	400	60	400	12
	19-22	120	5′4″	44	4,000	1.1	1.3	14	2.0	3.0	400	60	300	12
	23-50	120	5′4″	44	4,000	1.0	1.2	13	2.0	3.0	400	60	200	12
	51+	120	5′4″	44	4,000	1.0	1.2	13	2.0	3.0	400	60	200	12
Pregnant				+30	+1,000	+0.4	+0.3	+2	+0.6	+1.0	+400	+20	+200	+3.0
Lactating				+20	+2,000	+0.5	+0.5	+5	+0.5	+1.0	+100	+40	+200	+4.5

Minerals

	Age (yr.)	Weight (lb.)	Height	Calcium (mg.)	Iodine (mcg.)	Iron (mg.)	Magnesium (mg.)	Phosphorus (mg.)	Zinc (mg.)
All Women	11-14	101	5′2″	1,200	150	18	300	1,200	15
	15-18	120	5′4″	1,200	150	18	300	1,200	15
	19-22	120	5′4″	800	150	18	300	800	15
	23-50	120	5′4″	800	150	18	300	800	15
	51+	120	5′4″	800	150	10	300	800	15
Pregnant				+400	+25	30-60	+150	+400	+5
Lactating				+400	+50	30-60	+150	+400	+10

Estimated Safe and Adequate Daily Dietary Intakes for Other Minerals and Trace Elements

	Chloride (mg.)	Chromium (mg.)	Copper (mg.)	Fluoride (mg.)	Manganese (mg.)	Molybdenum (mg.)	Potassium (mg.)	Selenium (mg.)	Sodium (mg.)
All Women	1,700-5,100	0.05-0.20	2.0-3.0	1.5-4.0	2.5-5.0	0.15-0.50	1,875-5,625	0.05-0.20	1,100-3,300

SOURCE: *Recommended Dietary Allowances,* 9th ed. (Washington, D.C.: National Academy of Sciences, 1980).

toms associated with premenstrual syndrome. It's also been prescribed for women taking birth control pills, who often have lower blood levels of this vitamin. Mood changes, like depression, that are experienced by some women taking birth control pills have been attributed to lower levels of B_6, which some researchers speculate may lead to decreased production of the brain neurotransmitter serotonin. See your doctor if you think you need more than the RDA of B_6. High doses have been associated with neurological changes.

The Discriminating Mineral: Calcium

RDA charts list the same calcium requirement, 800 milligrams a day, for both men and women. This does not reflect the growing belief among nutritionists that women need more than this amount to prevent osteoporosis. Some feel that younger women need 1,000 milligrams and postmenopausal women up to 1,500 milligrams a day of calcium to help prevent this crippling disease of older women.

The problem is that many women don't get even 800 milligrams a day, Davis says. Calcium deficiencies among women are second only to iron deficiencies. The average intake for women is 600 milligrams

"Getting 1,000 milligrams a day of calcium means three or four servings of high-calcium foods, mostly dairy products," Davis says. "Although you can get this amount of calcium through foods—and that's the best way—it does take quite a bit of attention to do so without taking in a lot of calories." Low-fat dairy products or calcium supplements provide bone-building material without the fat-building side effects.

C H A P T E R

T W O

Customize Your Diet

Are you stressed? Pregnant? Using oral contraceptives? Exercising frequently? Such individual factors alter your nutritional needs. To keep your system supplied with everything it requires, here's a table to help you design a diet based on your personal lifestyle.

For each nutrient in the table, begin by reviewing the recommended intake levels that apply to "All Women." Then refer to the category or categories that apply to you—"Physically Active," "Dieters," "Stressed" and so forth. (In some cases, your needs for a nutrient may not change. For example, physically active women do not necessarily require more vitamin A or D than less active women.)

Who You Are, What You Need

Category	Vitamin A	Vitamin B	Vitamin C	Vitamin D
All Women	RDA = 4,000 I.U. Suggested optimum level = 5,000 I.U. The need for vitamin A increases with greater body weight.	RDA: thiamine = 1-1.1 mg.; riboflavin = 1.2-1.3 mg.; niacin = 13-14 mg.; B_6 = 2 mg.; folate = 400 mcg.; B_{12} = 3 mcg.; pantothenate = 4-7 mg.; biotin = 100-300 mcg. Suggested optimum levels: thiamine = 1.5-10 mg.; riboflavin = 5 mg.; niacin = 20-100 mg.; B_6 = 5-10 mg.; folate = 400 mcg.; B_{12} = 6 mcg.; pantothenate = 10 mg.; biotin = 300 mcg.	RDA = 60 mg. Suggested optimum level = 200-500 mg. Women who consume more than 90 mg. of vitamin C daily have been shown to cut their risk of cervical dysplasia in half.†	RDA = 200-300 I.U. Suggested optimum level = 400 I.U.
Physically Active		All B vitamins may be lost through perspiration. In a study at Cornell University, women who exercised vigorously for 30 to 50 minutes daily doubled their need for riboflavin.*†	Vitamin C plays a role in the formation of collagen, found in tendons, ligaments and muscles. Inadequate levels may cause fatigue.*	

Dieters	Low-calorie diets (1,200 calories or less) can reduce your intake of some or all nutrients, depending on the foods emphasized.	*	*	*
Stressed		Deficiencies of B vitamins have been shown to bring about such stress-related symptoms as nervousness, fatigue, depression, insomnia and headaches.*	Severe emotional stress may lower the plasma level of vitamin C.†	
Smokers	Research shows that vitamin A may somehow modify the cancer-causing effect of certain substances in the lung.†	Smoking can bring on a deficiency of B_{12} to detoxify the cyanide in cigarette smoke; the vitamin B_6 deficiency is possibly due to an interaction between this vitamin and carbon monoxide.*	Some researchers warn that smoking drains your body of 25 mg. of vitamin C per cigarette. Vitamin C can help detoxify carbon monoxide, cadmium, arsenic compounds and cyanide—all constituents of cigarette smoke.*†	

(continued)

Who You Are, What You Need—*Continued*

Category	Vitamin A	Vitamin B	Vitamin C	Vitamin D
City Dwellers (or exposed to pollution)	High intakes of vitamin A appear to protect against cancer. A vitamin A deficiency may increase the harmful effects of dangerous pollutants.† ‡		Vitamin C protects against more than 50 dangerous pollutants, including nitrates in food, ozone, cadmium, benzene, radiation and certain chemicals found in pesticides. (See Zinc.)‡	
Vegetarians		Riboflavin, vitamin B_{12} and folate levels may drop dangerously low.*		
Oral Contraceptive Users		Thiamine, riboflavin, B_6, folate and B_{12} may be depleted. Vitamin B_6 has been found to relieve depression in oral contraceptive users. Folate supplementation may reduce the risk of cervical cancer.*	Reduced body levels of vitamin C may exist. Vitamin C supplementation has been recommended.*‡	

Pregnant	RDA = 5,000 I.U.	RDA: thiamine = 1.4-1.5 mg.; riboflavin = 1.5-1.6 mg.; niacin = 15-16 mg.; B_5 = 2.6 mg.; folate = 800 mcg.; B_{12} = 4 mcg.; pantothenate = 4-7 mg. or more; biotin = 100-300 mcg. Folate and vitamin B_6 deficiencies are common. Folate supplementation may prevent serious spinal birth defects.*	RDA = 80 mg.	RDA = 400-500 I.U.
Lactating	RDA = 6,000 I.U.	RDA: thiamine = 1.5-1.6 mg.; riboflavin = 1.7-1.8 mg.; niacin = 18-19 mg.; folate = 500 mcg.; B_{12} = 4 mcg.; pantothenate = 4-7 mg.; biotin = 100-300 mcg. B_6 = 2.5 mg. Excessive doses of B_6 can reduce milk production, but supplements of up to 20 mg. per day are safe for lactating women and recommended to meet the infant's RDA.†	RDA = 100 mg.	RDA = 400-500 I.U.

(continued)

Who You Are, What You Need—*Continued*

Category	Vitamin A	Vitamin B	Vitamin C	Vitamin D
Cold & Flu Prone	The physical stress of illness can rob the body of up to 60 percent of its vitamin A. Large amounts are then needed to stimulate the immune response. In a slight deficiency, mucous membranes are weakened, making them more susceptible to viruses.*	Deficiencies of B_6, pantothenate and folate have been shown to seriously depress immunity.‡	Studies show that vitamin C increases resistance to infection. One tc 2 g. daily might be needed to stimulate the immune system.†	

Category	Vitamin E	Calcium	Iron	Zinc
All Women	RDA = 12 I.U.	RDA = 800 mg. Suggested optimum level = 1,000-1,300 mg.; 1,500 mg. for postmenopausal women. Research suggests that levels beyond the	RDA = 18 mg. Suggested optimum level = 18 mg. Forty percent of women age 20 to 50 show signs of iron deficiency. The average American diet	RDA = 15 mg. Suggested optimum level = up to 25 mg.

		RDA are needed by women as young as 20 to prevent osteoporosis, a bone-thinning condition that's common in the post-menopausal years.†	supplies only half the RDA for women.*	
Physically Active	Many athletes find that vitamin E improves aerobic capacity, muscle function and endurance.‡		Iron deficiency is common in athletic women, particularly during menstruation. Depletion of tissue iron may hurt performance even before blood iron dips to anemic levels.*	
Dieters	*	*	*	*
Stressed		Stress depletes calcium.*		
Smokers	Vitamin E decreases platelet aggregation, reducing the chances of blood clot formation in smokers.†	Smoking accelerates osteoporosis—the loss of calcium from the bones. To counteract this, extra doses of calcium are essential.*		

(continued)

Who You Are, What You Need—*Continued*

Category	Vitamin E	Calcium	Iron	Zinc
City Dwellers (or exposed to pollution)	Vitamin E may protect against damage caused by radiation, mercury, lead and two dangerous components of air pollution, nitrogen dioxide and ozone.‡	Calcium may protect against the accumulation of two toxic metals, cadmium and lead, in body tissues.‡	In laboratory animals, high levels of iron offered almost complete protection against cadmium toxicity.‡	Zinc and vitamin C may prevent the absorption of lead from the digestive tract and also help clear lead that's already been absorbed. Zinc may also block the accumulation of cadmium.‡
Vegetarians		Eliminating dairy products from the diet may lead to a calcium deficiency. Foods rich in C will promote calcium absorption.*	Blood iron in women can fall below optimum levels in some vegetarian diets.*	
Oral Contraceptive Users	Possible depletion.‡			Zinc levels in the blood may be reduced.*

Pregnant	RDA = 15 I.U.	RDA = 1,200 mg. Up to 1,600 mg. daily ensures the development of healthy bones in the fetus. Calcium also affects muscles, which may promote an easier delivery for the mother.†	RDA = 30-60 mg. A majority of women who become pregnant have partial or complete depletion of their iron reserves. Iron requirements increase in response to blood volume and the needs of the fetus, which, according to the National Academy of Sciences, cannot be met by existing body levels nor by diet. 30 to 60 mg. of ferrous salt should supplement an iron-rich diet.*	RDA = 20 mg.
Lactating	RDA = 16 I.U.	RDA = 1,200 mg. Women with a very high production of milk may need intakes much higher than the RDA.†	Iron needs for lactating women are the same as for nonpregnant women; however, it is recommended that supplementation of 30-60 mg. continue for two or three months after delivery to replenish stores depleted during pregnancy.*	RDA = 25 mg. In a recent study, the average zinc intake of lactating women was only 10.6 mg. At that level, the infants were receiving less than 50 percent of the RDA.*

(continued)

Who You Are, What You Need—*Continued*

Category	Vitamin E	Calcium	Iron	Zinc
Cold & Flu Prone	Vitamin E may stimulate antibody production and increase resistance to bacterial infections.‡		Iron, like zinc, is necessary for function of the white blood cells, which fight off infection.*	When even marginal amounts of dietary zinc are missing, the immune response quickly deteriorates.*

NOTE: Recommended nutrient levels are based on general information for average persons and should be considered as guidelines. For information specific to your own medical needs, consult a knowledgeable physician or registered dietitian.

*Depletion or deficiency may exist; take extra care to get adequate levels.

†Benefits have been demonstrated with higher supplemental intake, even in cases where nutrient levels were adequate.

‡There may be health benefits from this nutrient, but more research needs to be done. Information is based on limited animal studies or clinical experience.

C H A P T E R

T H R E E

Body Fat: A Better Measure of Fitness

It has taken more than a decade of research to confirm what fitness buffs already knew: Exercise not only improves your insides but enhances your outward appearance as well. For those who aspire to the body beautiful, working out has never had more proven advantages.

Chief among the pluses is exercise's power to shift your body's balance of fat and muscle. You already know that physical activity burns fat (and that in itself is a nice thing to note in the mirror), but you should also realize that working out increases muscle mass, too. This burning and building process changes your fat-to-muscle ratio, which in turn can alter how you look in a bathing suit.

You see, a pound of muscle is more densely packed than a pound of fat, so it's smaller. Thus a shift toward increased muscle and decreased fat can mean a slimmed-down appearance. A 135-pound woman, for example, could actually go down a dress size without losing a pound.

Muscle and fat don't just sit there and take up space—they use up calories. But muscle mass at rest burns more calories than fat does, which means that by adding muscle through exercise, you can increase your basal metabolic rate (the speed at which your body burns calories at rest) and thus hurry along the rate at which you shed extra pounds.

"Muscles are little furnaces that avidly metabolize food for energy," says Gabe Mirkin, M.D., author of the book *Getting Thin.* "Fat storage cells are exactly that—inert depots, for the most part."

Exercise is the only way you can *build* muscle mass while *decreasing* fat. Studies have shown that those who diet without exercise lose muscle first and fat second.

"With dieting alone, as much as 30 percent of the initial weight loss is muscle," says Ellen Coleman, exercise physiologist and director of the Riverside Cardiac Fitness Center in Riverside, California. "That probably explains why so many dieters look gaunt and saggy—they lose connective tissue along with fat. Exercise, on the other hand, burns fat while increasing muscle tone. So people who exercise to lose weight don't look saggy and wrinkled the way dieters do.

"People need to realize that appearance and percentage of body fat are the *real* measures of weight, not the numbers on their bathroom scale," says Coleman. "If not, they'll get discouraged and quit exercising. You can lose fat, gain muscle and weigh exactly the same. But you'll look thinner because your percentage of fat will be lower."

You'll not only look thinner—you'll *be* thinner. Take a tape measure to the newly muscular you. As you melt away the layer of fat beneath your skin, you'll melt away inch after inch of your thighs, hips, waist and other well-padded parts.

And *this* is exercise's greatest boon to womankind: Exercise ends the terrible tyranny of the scale. Who cares what you weigh? If you exercise, you look better, your clothes are looser and you feel prouder. Exercise offers you "a sense of accomplishment, self-esteem, well-being and self-control," asserts Konstantin N. Pavlou, Sc.D., a senior research associate in nutrition at Harvard Medical School.

How to Measure Your Body Fat

There are several ways to monitor your body fat and check your fitness progress. The most accurate method is done in an underwater tank. You are weighed first on a standard scale, then weighed again while immersed in water in a specially constructed tank. But to accurately measure body density, a necessary part of the body fat equation, a research assistant must determine how much air is in your lungs, as oxygen makes a body more buoyant. This is costly and time-consuming; expect to pay anywhere from $50 to $150 at fitness centers and university laboratories for this test.

Skinfold calipers are a more common method of measuring body fat. These spring-loaded pincers are inexpensive—some cost as little as $19.95 at pharmacies, medical supply outlets and mail-order sources. To use them properly, you'll need a partner to measure your body fat at four different sites. To ensure accuracy, have your partner take each measurement three or four times and record the average of the measurements at each test site.

The first measurement is the *bicep,* the muscle located in the front of the arm, midway between the elbow and the shoulder. Your partner should grab as much tissue as possible between his thumb and forefinger, then lift and pull it away from the bone and muscle underneath and take the measurement with the calipers. Next he should pinch and measure the *tricep,* the muscle found midway between the elbow and shoulder in the back of the arm. The next point, the *suprailiac,* is the muscle that runs diagonally along the right front portion of the hip. Place your index finger on your hipbone, with your thumb slightly above it, and pinch. Measure what you've grabbed with the calipers. Finally, have your partner pinch and measure along the *subcapular* muscle, which lies diagonally along the bottom of the "wing" bone in your back.

To arrive at your percentage of body fat, add up the averages of the four skinfold thickness measurements. Find that total in the lefthand column of the table on page 20, then read across under your age and sex group to find your body fat percentage. If information for your age group is not included in this table, use the table provided with your calipers, which may or may not require taking more measurements.

The body fat percentage you find in the table is the percentage of your total body weight that is made up of fat. For example, if you weigh 130 pounds and the measurements reveal that your body fat percentage is 25 percent, your body is composed of 97.5 pounds of muscle and bone mass and 32.5 pounds of fat. But if you weigh 130 pounds and your body fat percentage is 18 percent, your body is composed of 106.6 pounds of muscle and bone and only 23.4 pounds of fat. That's roughly 9 fewer pounds of fat, without "losing weight." The ideal percentage of body fat for women is 18 to 22 percent.

Calculating Your Body Fat Percentage

Skinfold Total (mm.)	Ages 16–29 (%)	Ages 30–49 (%)
14	9.4	14.1
16	11.2	15.7
18	12.7	17.1
20	14.1	18.4
22	15.4	19.5
24	16.5	20.6
26	17.6	21.5
28	18.6	22.4
30	19.5	23.3
35	21.6	25.2
40	23.4	26.8
45	25.0	28.3

NOTE: Figures apply to women only.

CHAPTER FOUR

Designing an Exercise Program That's Right for You

You're sold on the *idea* of fitness, but sticking to your workout schedule is another matter. It could be that your program is doomed to failure before your sneakers touch the ground, not because you lack will power but because you haven't found the exercises that suit you best.

Ten minutes in the locker room should be all it takes to prove to you once and for all that no two people, or bodies, are alike. Everyone has different strengths and problem areas—and different goals. To some, being fit means being able to run a good rat race; to others it means being able to run a good marathon.

So beware of exercise formulas that promise something for everybody. The only perfect program is the one that feels right for you, and the best way to find that one is to design it for yourself, based on your personal needs and goals.

What follows is a short course in customizing an exercise plan for yourself. No prescriptions. No directives. Just some advice on making getting fit more fun.

Rating Your Workouts

The benefits you derive from individual exercises will change as you progress through your fitness program. For example, the body toning you may notice as you progress as an ice skater will taper off once you get in the advanced league. At this point, the only thing you'll be improving is your aerobic fitness.

This table should give you an idea of the benefits you'll reap from some of the more popular forms of exercise, depending on your level of fitness. You can mix and match these workouts and custom-design a program that's most fun and beneficial for your personal needs.

Exercise	Aerobic Fitness	Flexi-bility	Toning	Strength
Aerobic dance	1, 2, 3		1, 2, 3	
Aqua aerobics	1, 2, 3	1, 2, 3	1	
Cross-country skiing	1, 2, 3			
Cycling	1, 2, 3		1, 2, 3	
Downhill skiing	3		2, 3	
Ice skating	1, 2, 3		1, 2	
Jogging/running	2, 3		2	
Martial arts		1, 2, 3	1, 2, 3	1
Racquetball	1, 2, 3		1, 2	
Rowing	1, 2, 3		1, 2, 3	
Swimming	1, 2, 3	1, 2, 3	1, 2, 3	
Tennis	2, 3		2, 3	
Walking/hiking	1		1, 2	
Yoga		1, 2, 3	1, 2	

NOTE: 1 = beginner; 2 = intermediate; 3 = advanced

Set Realistic Goals

What are your fitness goals? Do you want a flatter tummy? More muscle definition? Size 8 jeans? Extra energy to help you make it through a long working day? You've got to know your destination before you can decide how to get there. Setting objectives for yourself can give you a clearer idea of how to proceed with your fitness program and help you avoid wasting time on activities that aren't going to get you where you want to go. For example, if you're unhappy about a flabby stomach, tennis won't help you much, even if you play like a maniac. You need steady aerobic workouts to burn off the fat and Sit-Ups to tone your abdominal muscles.

But make sure your goals are simple and attainable. "Winning the Boston Marathon" is a goal that's likely to set you up for failure. But even a goal like "I will walk three blocks a day" is a step in the right direction. Keep your goals flexible so you can meet them reasonably well, despite unforeseen changes like injury, high-stress periods or bad weather.

The idea here is not to whip yourself into shape. That hurts. The point is to ease yourself into fitness. If you try to break world records right at the start, you are going to injure yourself—and get very discouraged awfully fast.

Lowell Scott Weil, D.P.M., a podiatrist from Des Plaines, Illinois, suggests that our body may know more about slow and easy fitness than we do. "Injuries often occur because people do not listen to the messages their own body sends them," he says. "They hear that exercise is painful, so when it begins to hurt, they push harder, when maybe they should stop. They forget that exercise involves regular but moderate demands placed on the body and its systems."

So forget that ridiculous philosophy that no pain means no gain. Be gentle with yourself. Try planning a realistic exercise quota for your first month and promise yourself a reward for reaching that short-term goal. You should be absolutely sure you can handle the quota—and up the ante only when you're positive you can handle the tougher challenge.

Reach for your own standards—not Jane Fonda's. Not Chris Evert Lloyd's. Not Joan Benoit Samuelson's. Exclude all external standards. That means crossing out "pleasing others." Exercise is, and should be, purely self-centered.

(continued on page 26)

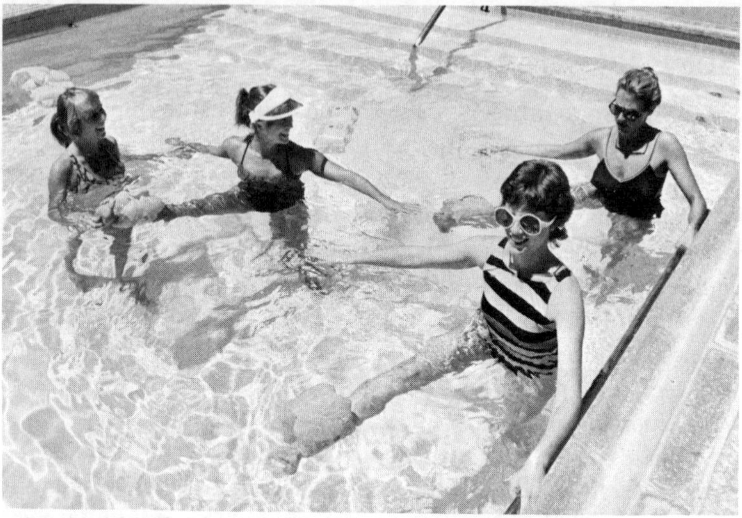

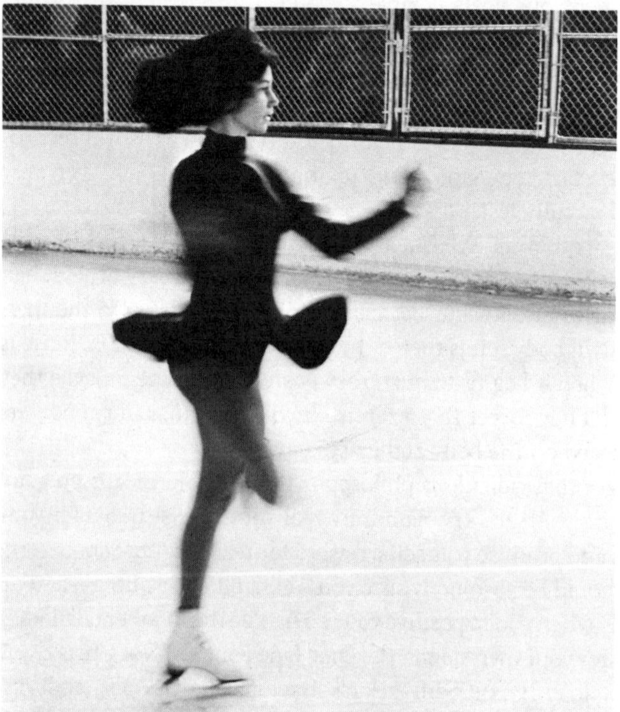

Aqua aerobics, ice skating, racquetball and tennis are some of the activities that can make getting fit fun.

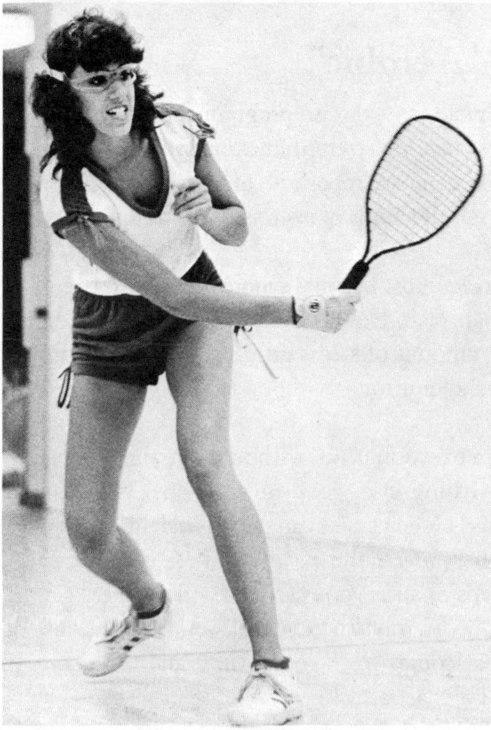

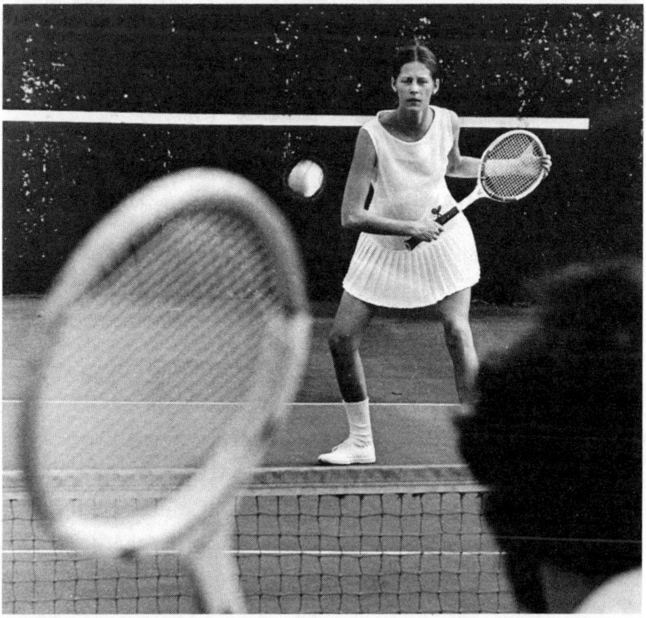

Do Something "Aerobic"

In order to be complete, an exercise program should emphasize each of three basic fitness factors: strength, flexibility and endurance. Endurance is probably the most important of the three, and it is achieved primarily through the kinds of exercises we've come to know as aerobic.

Aerobics classes have almost become synonymous with exercise. But aerobics is *more* than plain exercise. To be aerobic, an exercise must place a reasonable amount of stress on your heart and lungs. It must get you huffing and puffing—without stopping—for a good 30 minutes.

Of course, this extra exertion is not without its rewards. Aerobic exercise, better than anything else, gets you in shape. It gives you endurance. Your heart and blood vessels can more efficiently transport oxygen to the muscle cells, process the oxygen in those cells and carry off the waste. The rewards of such good cardiovascular fitness can be felt in every part of your body. You tire less easily, you get that sense of exuberant well-being that comes from good health and you decrease your chances of dying of a heart attack.

So how do you achieve this marvelous state? With repetitive, rhythmic exercise. One that makes use of your body's large muscles. One that gets your heart beating faster—significantly faster—so it can "idle" much slower when you're idle yourself. A friendly tennis game won't do it (too many pauses) unless you're fairly good at it—intermediate or advanced. Lifting weights, no matter how heavy they are, is not aerobic. Cycling's good if it makes you breathe hot and heavy, and if you don't spend half your time coasting. Jogging is dandy—no matter how slowly you go.

Researchers recommend raising the pulse rate during exercise to at least 70 or 80 percent of maximum. But how do you find 70 or 80 percent of your maximum? Simply use the number 220 as your absolute maximum pulse rate and then subtract your age from 220 to arrive at your age-adjusted maximum. For example, a 30-year-old would have an age-adjusted maximum of 190; 70 percent of that would be 133 beats per minute. However, it's important to keep in mind that none of this will do you any good unless you keep your pulse rate up for a good 30 minutes. And you should plan on exercising at that level *at least* three times a week.

Build a Strong Body

Strength training is an exercise program that involves working the muscles against gradually increasing degrees of resistance. It differs from exercises such as jogging and racquetball—which obviously also give your muscles a workout—by employing the "overload principle." That is, a conscious effort is made at several points in the workout to challenge the muscles with more resistance than they can comfortably handle for more than a few repetitions of the exercise. Muscles respond to the regular employment of overload challenges by steadily increasing in strength and sometimes in size as well.

What are the benefits of strength training to women? There are lots of benefits, it turns out. Benefits that can help all women—old, young and in between.

Greater strength is especially important to today's working woman. Many jobs in public safety, for instance, require that women pass the same strength and agility tests that men take. Businesswomen who must travel are at the mercy of cab drivers and porters unless they can carry a suitcase, a briefcase and a shoulder bag all at the same time for at least 15 minutes. And the self-defense courses women take can be pretty meaningless unless there's enough oomph behind that kick to get the point across. The weaker you are now, the more you stand to gain from strength training. One of the inevitable consequences of aging is a gradual loss of muscle mass. The result is that by the time you are over 40 or 50, your strength may be drastically less than it was at 20. By 65, a woman who has followed a sedentary lifestyle may have no more strength than a child. Fatigue comes easily, everyday tasks become monumental chores. Posture poops out, and you begin to think of yourself as old even though your mind may be as young as ever.

Strength training is just the ticket to combat this slide into premature senescence. While it's probably not possible for a person of 60 to maintain the same muscular strength he or she enjoyed at 20, it is definitely possible for a fit 60-year-old to enjoy the strength of the average 45-year-old or for a 45-year-old to have the power of a 25-year-old.

If you have never followed a strength-building program before, you can actually *reverse* muscle deterioration by starting one now. You'll be building muscle instead of losing it. As each day passes and you continue your workouts, your muscles will in effect become younger and younger. Eventually you'll reach a limit to this rejuvenating effect, but by that time you'll be well ahead of the game. It may never have occurred to you that muscles are built-in safety pads, but orthopedic surgeons know it all too well. A person with very little muscle mass between skin and bone to absorb the shock of a fall or other potentially serious injury is that much more likely to suffer a broken or severely bruised bone. A strong arm, quickly extended, may prevent the impact from occurring in the first place, or at least reduce its severity. These two protective functions are important at any age, but they become increasingly valuable protection to anyone who wants to pursue an active lifestyle as long as possible.

Strength is beautiful. Not just in the metaphorical sense of making you more energetic and self-reliant, but in the most literal sense as well. We are talking about arms and legs that don't look like they've had their vital substance sucked out. We are talking about shoulders that don't slump, posture that doesn't sag. We're talking about strong abdominal muscles that hold your stomach and intestines behind your belt without any artificial restraint.

No matter where you look, good muscles look good.

Stretch, Tone and Flex

Flexibility is crucial to health. Scientists define flexibility as the "range of motion about a joint"—how far you can reach, turn, twist, swing and bend. As we grow older, flexibility declines. We become tight, creaky, limited. Aging itself could be seen as a gradual decrease in flexibility. Staying flexible means we can stay supple, loose—and young.

To improve flexibility, stretch. A study at the University of Oregon showed that women who did routine stretching exercises became significantly more limber. And those who were considered in "average" shape at the beginning of the semester-long experiment made the greatest gains. A similar study at the University of Iowa found that women who took part in daily stretching exercises for three weeks improved substantially in virtually all flexibility tests.

To further improve mobility, warm up with a few minutes of light calisthenics, jogging in place or slow cycling before you work out. Even a single preliminary movement, a Toe Touch, for example, results in a better score for that test. *Research Quarterly* reported a study involving 33 college men who were tested in the Toe Touch over a five-week period. Men who practiced the Toe Touch and other exercises before the test did considerably better than men who started cold. Another study with high school students and adults tested 20 joint movements and found that all 20 tests improved with warm-up. That's why athletes do stretching exercises before competing. They don't waste energy; they improve performance.

Don't reach beyond your grasp: there is no such thing as "normal" flexibility. The range of natural movement varies greatly from person to person. You can admire the person who can touch his toes with his elbows, but you don't have to be able to do it to be in the same physical shape.

You should try to loosen up *all* of you, not just your back or legs. Take note if some parts of your body seem to be more flexible than others. Flexibility in one joint doesn't guarantee equal range of motion in other body parts.

Incidentally, one of the oldest myths in the world of fitness and sports is that weight training causes a "muscle-bound" condition that limits an athlete's ability to move. Research has proven just the opposite. One study found that body builders who achieved international recognition in physique competitions and weight trainers who took part in weight-lifting events generally had greater flexibility than normal groups of 16-year-old boys. Another study found that in a speed test that required members of a university weight-lifting team and a control group of students to turn a crank at high speed, the weight lifters had arm movement speed equal to that of the other group.

C H A P T E R

F I V E

Gyn-Ecology: Keeping Vaginal Infections in Check

Despite all the high-technology advances in obstetrics and gynecology, yeast infections and other vaginal conditions continue to plague us at an unrelenting pace. Why?

Sexual freedom is one reason: The more partners a woman has, the greater her risk of exposure to infectious organisms. (For more information on sexually transmitted diseases, see chapter 9.) But there's another, more important, reason—body ecology.

Whether or not an infection is sexually transmitted, it's the climate, or ecological balance, within the vagina—or neighboring urinary tract—that largely determines the course it will take. A healthy environment is hostile to invading organisms and can usually fight off a minor assault. An imbalance in the ecosystem, however, can create an environmental haven for troublesome bacteria, viruses and fungi.

Unfortunately, there are many factors that can disrupt the gyn-ecological balance. Before we learn what they are, let's take a look at how this ecosystem really works.

Your Natural Defense System

Under normal conditions, the vagina is host to a variety of microorganisms that may include *Staphylococcus* (the bacterium associated with toxic shock syndrome) and *Escherichia coli* (the predominant cause of urinary tract infections). To keep these potentially threatening organisms in check, there is also an assortment of beneficial bacteria such as *Lactobacillus* and Döderlein's bacillus.

The *Lactobacilli* are largely responsible for maintaining the vagina's slightly acidic pH at about 4.5 or below (on a scale of 0 to 14, in which 7 is neutral). Trichomoniasis, gardnerella and other infectious organisms require a pH of 5 or above in order to thrive.

If it weren't for the *Lactobacilli,* the vagina might always be a sugary, alkaline breeding ground for infections. That's because the cells of the vaginal walls store sugar in the form of glucose; vaginal secretions slough off the cells, releasing the glucose.

Bacteria, fungi and protozoa love to feed off sugar. The *Lactobacilli* thrive on sugar, too, but unlike the other organisms, the *Lactobacilli* convert the sugar into lactic acid. This mild acid kills off many of the offending organisms.

Another important protective system is the cervical mucus, an odorless discharge that fluctuates between a clear egg-white consistency and a milky-white paste, depending on where you are in your menstrual cycle.

Glands located in the cervix secrete this mucus, which bathes the vagina, washing away debris and cells naturally shed from the vaginal walls. "Merely wiping the lips of the vagina is then sufficient to cleanse the cavity," explains Gideon G. Panter, M.D., a New York City gynecologist and faculty member at New York Hospital-Cornell Medical Center.

The mucus has other important functions. It moistens and lubricates the vaginal walls, thereby protecting them from damage. And mucus "plugs" the cervical opening, preventing the spread of infection to the uterus and fallopian tubes, where it could result in the fertility-threatening condition known as pelvic inflammatory disease (PID).

Disrupting the Gyn-Ecological Balance

Of course, there are all kinds of conditions that can make you more—or less—susceptible to infection.

Stress, anxiety and lack of sleep can lower immunity and may even increase vaginal alkalinity, making you vulnerable to all kinds of infections.

Your menstrual cycle also affects your vulnerability. Cervical mucus is slightly more alkaline when you're most fertile. And during menstruation, the blood that floods the vagina serves as a sweet, alkaline medium—which is why many women find that their yeast infection or trichomoniasis symptoms escalate during or after their periods.

The timing of sex during the menstrual cycle can further aggravate this effect. For example, the combination of semen and menstrual blood forms a superfertile medium for bacterial growth. And with the cervix slightly dilated during menstruation, there's an increased chance for upward movement of bacteria into the uterine cavity and the development of pelvic inflammatory disease.

During pregnancy, vaginitis becomes an even greater threat due to the hormonal changes that cause more sugar to be stored in the vaginal cells, increasing alkalinity. The Pill can have the same effect.

Antibiotic use is another factor. Ironically, antibiotics are often prescribed for vaginal infections caused by certain types of bacteria. The problem is that in the process of wiping out the bad guys, the antibiotics kill off the good bacteria—the *Lactobacilli*—that keep the vagina acidic. That's why many women find themselves plagued with yeast infections following antibiotic treatment.

Dietary Links

The foods you eat affect your body's ecology, too. Simple carbohydrates and sugars—pastries, hot fudge sundaes, even wine and cocktails—may make you more prone to vaginal infections, particularly yeast infections.

Though the link has never been scientifically proven, many women and women's health-care practitioners agree that cutting out sugar cuts down infections. And the connection makes sense: Diabetes, pregnancy and the Pill all increase the amount of sugar that's stored in the vaginal walls, and they have been known to trigger yeast infections. It's not that difficult to understand, then, how a diet high in sugar might have similar consequences.

There's yet another dietary link to vaginitis: Some doctors believe that fungus-related foods may encourage *Candida,* the fungus that causes yeast infections.

Candida is biologically related to molds in cheese and to yeast in beer, wine, vinegar and breads. Eating these foods may overload the system with molds or yeasts, which can cause a yeast infection to flare. (Other yeast-containing foods include breaded meat, fish and chicken; buttermilk; malt-flavored milk drinks; sour cream; mushrooms; sauerkraut; dried fruit; frozen or canned citrus juice; root beer; ginger ale; horseradish; soy sauce; pickles; and B vitamins made from yeast.)

Incidentally, some livestock are fed antibiotics—which, of course, can trigger yeast infections. You might want to try a meat-free diet or stick with organically grown meat if you're prone to yeast infections.

Some people may actually eat their way into recurrent herpes episodes when they choose foods containing a high amount of arginine, one of the amino acids. Scientists have found that arginine supports the growth and reproduction of the herpes virus. Foods high in arginine include nuts (almonds, cashews and peanuts), grains (wheat, barley and oats), corn, chocolate and coconut.

On the other hand, lysine, another amino acid, has been found to inhibit the growth of the virus by lessening the amount of arginine the body absorbs during digestion.

Jonathan Wright, M.D., of Kent, Washington, who specializes in nutritional treatment, explains that the ratio of arginine to lysine in foods is critical. If a food has a high arginine-to-lysine ratio, it could set off herpes. Foods that have a higher lysine-to-arginine ratio could help cut herpes episodes short. Meat, potatoes, milk and brewer's yeast contain a large proportion of lysine.

The results of experiments using lysine dietary supplements have been mixed. Various researchers have reported that dosages of from 500 to 1,000 milligrams a day help lessen pain and heal the herpes lesions faster. But some studies that used control groups given placebos were less than promising. You may want to experiment on your own to see whether lysine helps, since the effective dosages are harmless.

The Sweet Smell of Disaster

Perhaps the most blatant contributors to vaginal infections are soaps, scented bubble baths and feminine hygiene products. These can throw your ecosystem completely out of kilter. One study found a higher incidence of vulvovaginitis (inflammation of the vulva and vagina) among women who used bubble baths, feminine deodorant

(continued on page 39)

A Guide to Symptoms and Treatments of Gynecological Infections

Name	Classification	Symptoms	Your Course of Action	Medical Diagnosis and Treatment	Important Facts
Candidiasis or Monilia (commonly called yeast infection)	Fungus	Red, itchy vulva. Creamy, curdy discharge, burning on urination. Painful intercourse. Bright red vagina with white patches on walls and cervix.	Insert boric acid nightly. Or rub monistat or Gyne-Lotrimin cream on the vulva three times a day; place a single "shot" in the vagina at night. Yeast-free diet; acidophilus supplements. Salt-water baths. See a medical professional after 1 week.	Diagnosis: Wet-mount smear; immediate results. Treatment: Antifungal creams and suppositories like nystatin, monistat, miconazole, clotrimazole, imidazole, Gentian violet.	Can damage vaginal walls, making them more susceptible to invasion by other bacteria. Newborns infected through vaginal delivery can get oral infection, which interferes with nursing.
Chlamydia	Intermediate organism (neither bacteria nor virus)	Thin, white discharge. Painful intercourse; bleeding after intercourse. Burning on urination. Fever, chills, vomiting. Abdominal, back, leg or	See a medical professional immediately.	Diagnosis: Blood test now available (immunofluorescent); results in 4 hours. Culture tests also used but take several days for results. Treatment: Orally administered antibiotics like	Highly contagious. Can lead to pelvic inflammatory disease (PID). Infected newborns can develop serious eye infections and pneumonia.

		pelvic pain. No symptoms appear in early stages in 75% of cases.		tetracycline, sulfonamide, erythromycin.	
Gardnerella (sometimes called *Hemophilus vaginalis* or nonspecific vaginitis)	Bacteria	Red, itchy vulva. Light discharge that looks and feels like flour paste (gray-white and sticky) and has a strong fishy odor. Painful urination and intercourse.	Saltwater bath before bed for 3 nights. See a medical professional if symptoms persist.	Diagnosis: Wet-mount smear; immediate results. "Whiff test": exposure of vaginal secretions to drop of 10% KOH solution yields characteristic fishy smell. Immediate but not definitive results. Treatment: Orally administered antibiotics like ampicillin. Use of sulfa vaginal cream, Keflex, Flagyl.	Not serious but very annoying. Highly contagious. Responsible for most infections previously labeled nonspecific vaginitis.
Gonorrhea	Bacteria	Thin, white discharge. A thicker discharge may cling to cervix. Burning on urination. Pelvic pain. Symptoms may be subtle. Often confused with other conditions.	See a medical professional immediately.	Diagnosis: Culture; results in 2 days. Treatment: Penicillin injections or oral antibiotics such as ampicillin, amoxicillin or tetracycline.	Can lead to pelvic inflammatory disease (PID). May cause blindness in babies if transmitted during birth.

(continued)

A Guide to Symptoms and Treatments of Gynecological Infections—*Continued*

Name	Classification	Symptoms	Your Course of Action	Medical Diagnosis and Treatment	Important Facts
Herpes Simplex Type II	Virus	Clusters of small, painful or itchy blisters on genitals, buttocks or thighs, usually accompanied by local swelling. Fever, aching muscles and swollen glands in groin. Burning on urination. Recurrent infections may diminish in severity. Recurrences often start with itching, tingling, aching or burning at site of eventual outbreak.	Keep lesion clean and dry. Apply alcohol, peroxide or witch hazel directly to sore with cotton swab. Topical anesthetics like Lidocaine may ease pain. Ice packs help swelling and discomfort. Warm baths with Epsom salts or baking soda can be soothing. Urination in a bathtub filled with water may help if otherwise painful. Supplement diet with lysine. See a medical professional before blisters break.	Diagnosis: Culture grown from tissue scraped from base of open blister (only definitive measure). Blood test. Frequently misdiagnosed. Treatment: New antivirals (acyclovir, Adenine arabinoside) seem topically effective in primary attacks and only when used early in course of infection. Major drawbacks to these in present form (cream, ointment) is that they keep lesion moist. However, a 5-day course of acyclovir treatment may prevent new lesion formation and shorten healing time in recurrent episodes.	More than half of sufferers will never have second attack. Recurrence is related to general health—emotional, physical and strength of body's resistance. Creams containing cortisone should be avoided; they slow healing and may cause spread of virus. Women should be monitored carefully during pregnancy; virus can seriously affect infant infected by active lesion during birth. A statistical link has also been established between cancer of the cervix and genital herpes, although researchers have not found that herpes causes cervical cancer. If you contract herpes, it's a good idea to follow up with a Pap smear every 6 to 12 months.

Pelvic Inflammatory Disease (PID)	Various causes	Earliest symptoms often go undetected. Pain on one or both sides of abdomen. Chills. Vaginal discharge (bloody or puslike). Burning on urination. Painful intercourse. Nausea, vomiting.	See a medical professional immediately.	Diagnosis: Culture for gonorrhea and/or chlamydia (more accurate than routine aerobes/anaerobes test). Treatment: Oral antibiotics like tetracycline, penicillin and Flagyl. Hospitalization may be required.	Serious health problem. May be caused by bacterial or intermediate organisms that have migrated to the pelvic cavity. Misdiagnosed in one-third of all cases. Can cause salpingitis (infection of the fallopian tubes), which may promote sterility or increase likelihood of tubal pregnancy. Also responsible for endometriosis, cysts, abscesses.
Trichomoniasis	Protozoa	Vagina and vulva look wet and inflamed. Discharge that may be heavy, itchy, foamy, irritating, bad smelling and greenish yellow in color. Lower abdominal pain. Painful intercourse. Tendency to worsen after menstruation. Frequent urination.	Saltwater bath before bed for 3 nights. See a medical professional if symptoms persist after several days.	Diagnosis: Culture; results in 5 days. Wet-mount smear; immediate results. (Only definitive for positive results.) Pap smear. Treatment: Flagyl is only sure cure. New research indicates 1 large dose as effective as 7-day treatment and has fewer side effects.	Can cause changes in cervical cells that may increase chances of more serious cervical disease later on.

(continued)

A Guide to Symptoms and Treatments of Gynecological Infections—*Continued*

Name	Classification	Symptoms	Your Course of Action	Medical Diagnosis and Treatment	Important Facts
Urinary Tract Infections (caused by a variety of organisms, including *E. coli.* Usually referred to by site rather than type of infection.)	Bacteria	Uncomfortable and almost continual need to urinate. Burning on urination and sometimes blood in urine. Low abdominal pain, backache. Pain with intercourse. In more serious cases, chills, fever, lack of appetite, vomiting and pain in the kidneys.	Drink lots of water, at least 8 glasses a day (enough to make urine colorless). Cranberry juice is a good substitute because acid in it inhibits bacterial growth. Avoid coffee and tea. See a medical professional if symptoms persist for 24 hours.	Diagnosis: Laboratory analysis of urine sample to identify bacterial agent. Treatment: Antibiotics.	Annoying and inconvenient but not a threat to general health. If untreated, infection can spread to kidneys.

SOURCES: Adapted from *Healthy Sex and Keeping It That Way,* by Richard Lumiere and Stephani Cook (New York: Simon & Schuster, 1983).
"How to Deal with Sexually Transmitted Diseases," by Michael Castleman, *Medical Self-Care,* Spring 1983.
The American Medical Association Family Medical Guide, Jeffrey R. M. Kunz, ed. (New York: Random House, 1982).
Better Homes and Gardens New Family Medical Guide, Edwin Kiester, Jr., ed. (Des Moines: Meredith, 1982).
Take Care of Yourself, by Donald Vickery and James Fries (Reading, Mass.: Addison-Wesley, 1981).
Medical Self-Care and Assessment, by Brent Q. Hafen (Englewood, Colo.: Morton, 1983).

NOTE: Check with your practitioner about drug side effects and interactions. Pregnant women should be cautious of all oral medications and avoid Flagyl, podophyllin, some antifungal agents and some antibiotics, especially tetracycline. Nursing mothers should avoid Flagyl.

sprays and douches. The feminine hygiene sprays were the worst offenders.

Deodorant tampons and napkins can cause similar irritation. Deodorant tampons are an especially worthless idea, because menstrual blood has no odor until it's exposed to air.

Douching is bad for several reasons: You can have an allergic reaction to the chemicals that go into perfumed, commercially prepared douches. Douching also dries out the protective mucus and can irritate or damage the vaginal walls and upset the acid balance.

Worse, improper douching can propel microorganisms from the vagina into the uterus and even beyond if it's done at too high a pressure. Frequent douching can erode the mucus plug that acts as a protective barrier to the uterus and fallopian tubes.

It's particularly inadvisable to douche during menstruation or pregnancy or when the cervix is dilated and the upward flow can bring infected material to the uterus.

What to Wear

The dark, damp atmosphere in the vagina can also encourage the breeding of infectious organisms. This has led more than one physician and self-help center to recommend cotton underwear or panty shields to absorb excess moisture. But Marilynne McKay, M.D., of Emory University's School of Medicine, disagrees. Panty shields may increase perspiration, and the plastic backing on many of the liners blocks moisture, she says, thereby encouraging the growth of microorganisms. Contrary to popular belief, cotton underwear also holds moisture and may even be worse than nylon or synthetics, she adds.

Fortunately, Formfit Rogers makes a line of panties called Lita, made of a fabric containing the same propylene fiber used in workout wear. According to the company, Lita "breathes" and sheds moisture better than either nylon or cotton, so the skin stays dry and comfortable.

If, despite these precautions, you fall victim to an infection, don't give up. Keep in mind that by *restoring* your gynecological balance you may help speed your body's response to medical treatment or even stop an invasion early enough to save yourself a trip to the doctor's office. Being mindful of your body's ecology will give you an important edge in fighting back.

C H A P T E R

S I X

Simple Steps to Stop Cystitis

Urination is something you take for granted—until the urine burns like iodine on a raw wound. Or until you feel like you have to "go" right after you've just "gone." Your abdomen and back ache. You may even pass a drop or two of blood.

Cystitis, a urinary tract infection, affects millions of people—mostly women. And it's generally not a once-in-a-lifetime experience. In 80 percent of those who get cystitis, the infection returns again and again. Each time, they're awakened several times a night by the urge to urinate. They run to the bathroom every 20 minutes at work, and often they are in too much pain to concentrate on their job. On a personal level, they no longer enjoy sexual relations.

Cystitis may be caused by any of various organisms, including *Trichomonas* and *Chlamydia.* The most common cause, though, is *Escherichia coli* bacteria, which normally live in the large intestine and the rectum without causing any trouble. If those bacteria find their way into the urethra—the 1½-inch-long tube leading to the bladder and kidneys—the resulting infection makes urination urgent, frequent and

Symptoms of Cystitis

According to Larrian Gillespie, M.D., the signs of cystitis are easy to recognize:

- The urgent need to urinate often.
- Sharp stinging during urination, often accompanied by a gnawing pain in the lower abdomen.
- Occasionally, blood in the urine.
- A feeling that the bladder is full, even after urination.

Recognizing the illness can hasten relief of cystitis.

painful. Should the infection spread to the kidneys—a rare occurrence—it can do serious damage.

Certainly it's only a tiny trip from the rectum to the urethra, but certain habits make that trip even easier for bacteria to take. Sexual activity seems to trigger recurrent cystitis in women. The theory is that intercourse pushes bacteria from the area of the urethra into the bladder. Simply washing before and after sex helps to sanitize the area and prevent infection. Another preventive measure is to urinate within ten minutes after sex, thus flushing bacteria and other organisms out of the urethra before they have a chance to do their dirty work.

Preventive Hygiene

Still, women of all ages, from little girls to elderly widows, get cystitis, so there's clearly more to recurrent cystitis than sex. Wiping from back to front after a bowel movement drags rectal bacteria into the urethral opening. The reverse—wiping from front to back—prevents that.

No matter how busy you are, don't hold your urine indefinitely after feeling the urge. Ignoring nature's call distends the bladder wall, making it more susceptible to infection. And when urine accumulates in the bladder, so does bacteria. An empty bladder is less readily infected.

Wearing loose clothing and cotton underwear also helps to prevent cystitis. Tight jeans, girdles, panty hose and nylon briefs "hermetically seal" and irritate the urethral area, contributing to the growth of bacteria.

Women are especially prone to cystitis during pregnancy, particularly during the last three months. At that time, organs are crowded together. Scrunched between the womb and the pubic bone, the bladder may not be able to empty completely. Bacteria lingering in leftover urine become fruitful and multiply. During pregnancy, it's especially important to take precautions against cystitis, because hormonal changes at that time seem to encourage susceptibility.

Women who use a diaphragm for birth control may find it increases susceptibility to infection. The device's rim can push against the neck of the bladder, preventing complete urination. Changing to either a slightly smaller diaphragm or another method of birth control prevented further bouts of cystitis in 98.4 percent of women studied by Larrian Gillespie, M.D., a urologist and clinical instructor at the University of California at Irvine.

C H A P T E R

S E V E N

A Troubleshooting Guide to Menstrual Maladies

Sometime during your reproductive years, you're bound to experience a problem with your period. You could have something as minor as a delay in flow or as menacing as many missed periods. Depending upon your age, history and habits, it may simply be a side effect of too much exercise, or it could be a clue to a serious problem like uterine cancer.

Whatever your symptoms, though, menstrual irregularities usually occur when the hormones estrogen and progesterone are out of balance and ovulation becomes irregular.

Younger women usually experience more menstrual disturbances like missed or skipped periods (called amenorrhea). That means they are not ovulating. And women who have gained body fat or lost it (frequently from strenuous exercise) may have an altered estrogen output, which can stop their periods.

Women in their thirties and forties, on the other hand, are more likely to have midcycle problems, like breakthrough bleeding or a change in flow patterns. That's because the ovaries are aging and

(continued on page 46)

Defining Problem Periods

Problem	Probable Causes
Too many periods (less than 22 days apart)	Failure to ovulate; egg may not be completing luteal phase in ovary; thyroid disturbances; hormone imbalance; stress.
Too few periods (more than 35 days apart)	Failure to ovulate; may be preparing for menopause; excessive exercise, reduced red meat intake; stress; hormone imbalance.
Missed or no periods	Discontinuing the Pill; low body fat from vegetarian diet or excessive exercise; stress; thyroid disturbances; extreme eating disorders; hypothalamus dysfunctions; endocrine problems; ovarian cysts; medications such as amphetamines and tranquilizers.
Heavy flow	Intrauterine device (IUD); anemia; pelvic inflammatory disease; miscarriage; polyps; fibroids and cysts; abortion complications; in older women, may be a symptom of uterine cancer.
Light flow	Increased exercise; reduced red meat intake.
Prolonged flow	IUD-related; anemia; tubal pregnancy; underactive thyroid; fibroids; polyps; may be a symptom of uterine cancer.

Breakthrough bleeding (spotting between periods)	May be related to normal ovulation or temporary lack of estrogen at ovulation; lack of ovulation; infection; birth control pills; tubal pregnancy; polyps; fibroids; vaginal infections.
Clotting	Associated with heavy flow and cramping; miscarriage.
Bleeding after menopause (after periods stopped for 8 months)	Polyps; infection; injury as result of vaginal dryness and wall thinning; may be symptom of uterine, vaginal, cervical or vulvar cancer.
Bleeding after intercourse	Injury to existing lesions; polyps; herpes of the cervix or vagina; vaginal abrasions from fingernails, tampons; infection from partner; may be sign of syphilis of the cervix.
Severe cramps (often accompanied by nausea, vomiting, diarrhea, headache, backache)	Onset of menstruation (primary dysmenorrhea); benign uterine tumors (polyps, fibroids); pelvic infections; endometriosis; IUD insertion (secondary dysmenorrhea).

starting to shrink, and the blood supply is being interrupted. Major menstrual irregularities in older and postmenopausal women may signal a serious problem.

If the cause of your menstrual problem is minor and you have intermittent bleeding, your health-care provider may advise you to get more rest, reduce your exercise regimen and modify your diet with plenty of vegetables and foods rich in protein, B_{12}, magnesium and folate. Excessive bleeding problems may respond to nonsteroidal anti-inflammatory drugs such as ibuprofen, which is available by prescription as Motrin or over the counter as Advil or Nuprin, among others. Iron supplements may be recommended to combat anemia. Progesterone hormones may also be prescribed to stabilize fluctuating estrogen levels.

In other cases, menstrual disturbances may require further diagnostic procedures to pinpoint problems caused by cysts, uterine cancer, fibroid tumors, endometriosis or pelvic inflammatory disease. Surgery may be suggested to treat these problems, so be sure to seek a second opinion to ask about alternative treatments.

The table on pages 44 and 45 can give you some idea of what may be the cause of menstrual problems. In some cases, a medical exam is the only way to pinpoint the exact problem and decide on treatment.

CHAPTER EIGHT

Protect Your Breasts

The breast, for all its functional and ornamental attributes, is vulnerable to some very uncomfortable and worrisome ailments, the most alarming of which is cancer. Confusion over risk factors and mass screening for breast cancer, combined with blazing headlines that 1 out of every 13 women faces breast cancer each year, can prompt you to react in either of two ways: you nervously devour all the facts and theories and pray that you never have trouble, or else you throw up your hands in utter hopelessness.

Those same hands, however, can easily be educated to examine your own breasts for abnormalities and thereby help to minimize your chances of becoming a cancer statistic. Early detection *can* save your life. While doctors maintain that breast self-examination (BSE) is the single most important action you can take against breast cancer, BSE does not *prevent* cancer. However, some promising new studies are focusing on what does prevent cancer. Based on the findings, it's now estimated, for example, that breast cancer could be reduced by a full 50 percent with changes in our diet.

What are the components of an anti-breast cancer diet? And are there any other preventive actions we can take? The answers to these questions form the basis of the following recommendations.

Reduce Dietary Fats

In recent years, researchers have found a strong parallel between fat consumption and the incidence of breast cancer. Countries like Japan and Thailand, where low-fat diets are the rule, have only about one-quarter the number of breast cancer deaths that occur in the United States, Denmark and the Netherlands, where people consume up to twice as much fat.

These data are backed up by more than 25 years of animal studies that provide overwhelming evidence that a high-fat diet encourages the development of breast tumors. Indeed, some scientists believe that the data linking the two is nearly as convincing as the evidence linking smoking with lung cancer.

The question is, why?

According to Sherwood L. Gorbach, M.D., and Margo Woods, D.Sc., professors of medicine at Tufts University School of Medicine and authors of *The Doctor's Anti-Breast Cancer Diet,* the reason most likely has to do with the fat/estrogen connection. It's been known for some time that high estrogen levels increase a woman's vulnerability to breast cancer. What the Tufts professors found in their own research was that women who eat more meat (and more fat) excrete less estrogen in their stools and have higher estrogen levels in their bloodstream than vegetarians.

Other studies have shown that some women's bodies convert cholesterol into estrogen, and still others suggest that the cholesterol acts directly on breast tissue. Surplus fat and cholesterol may also lower the body's immunity.

Whatever the mechanism, the advice of Dr. Gorbach and Dr. Woods is to reduce all fat—not just saturated fat—from its present level (about 40 percent of total caloric intake) to 30 percent or, preferably, 25 percent. To give you a better idea of what this means: As a typical American woman with a daily intake of approximately 1,800 calories, you are probably consuming the fat equivalent of 6 tablespoons of butter a day. To reduce your breast cancer risk, your total fat intake should be closer to 3½ tablespoons of butter a day.

To move closer to your target fat intake, try to limit your red meat intake to two or three servings a week. Eat more chicken (preferably skinless breasts), fish and vegetarian dishes. Use butter, margarine and vegetable oils sparingly. Avoid eggs and choose low-fat or nonfat dairy products.

Increase Fiber Intake

There is less scientific evidence to support the role dietary fiber plays in the prevention of breast cancer, but studies to date do point in this direction. Dr. Gorbach and Dr. Woods explain that, according to their research, fiber was the second favorable component of a vegetarian diet. The vegetarian women in the study ate about 30 percent less fat than their meat-eating counterparts, and because of the high fiber content of their diets, their fecal output was nearly three times greater. This no doubt helped to flush the estrogen from the body, they say.

Another study confirms this association: Researchers at the University of California at San Francisco found that women with severe constipation (two or fewer bowel movements a week) were five times more likely to show signs of possible abnormal cell proliferation in fluids aspirated from their breasts than were women with normal bowel function.

"It may be that estrogen secreted by the liver is reabsorbed more readily by women with sluggish digestion," says Nicholas Petrakis, M.D., professor of preventive medicine at the University of California at San Francisco. "This could have a stimulating effect on breasts."

Fortunately, with the exception of nuts, most high-fiber foods are also low in fat. So, to the extent that you can move your diet in the direction of high-fiber foods, you'll gain two clear advantages. Some suggestions: Eat a high-fiber cereal for breakfast every day; snack on fresh fruits and vegetables; switch to whole grain breads and brown rice; and try to incorporate more beans, legumes and whole grains into your soups, salads and main courses. Incidentally, beans also contain substances called protease inhibitors that may block the cancer-causing process.

Eat Foods High in Vitamins A, C and E and Selenium

While the final verdict is not yet in on the cancer-inhibiting effect of vitamin A, there's a tremendous amount of interest in its potential. "The data from animal studies is quite encouraging," says Marc Lippman, M.D., director of the breast cancer division of the National Institutes of Health.

Maurice Black, M.D., of the Institute of Breast Disease of the New York Medical College, is using short-term high oral doses of both vitamins A and E in women who have had one incidence of breast cancer. This study arose out of another, related study of immunity and tumor growth that identified patients who seemed to be less resistant to tumors. Those patients participated in the high-dose vitamin studies.

These women don't naturally show the kind of immune response associated with good survival rates, Dr. Black says. But with large doses of either A or E, 50 to 60 percent do show this immune response. With *both* A and E, 80 percent show the response. "We don't yet know if this induced response works as well as a spontaneous response," Dr. Black says. "We haven't been following these women long enough to see if they have a reduced incidence of recurrent and/or second primary breast cancer."

Vitamin C is another nutrient that's been showing much promise on the cancer front. Although no study has correlated vitamin C intake specifically with breast cancer, it is known that this vitamin plays a protective role in numerous other cancers and viral illnesses. Like vitamins A and E, C is a potent antioxidant. That is, it defends cell membranes against the assault of free radicals, highly unstable molecules that can scramble the genetic information in a cell, starting a chain reaction that can lead to cancer. Vitamin C is also known to stimulate the immune system.

Selenium seems to have a protective effect as well. "The results of animal and human population studies continue to be encouraging that the risk of breast cancer does decline if selenium intakes are high," says Gerhard Schrauzer, Ph.D., professor of chemistry at the University of California at San Diego. In mice bred to carry a virus that puts them at high risk of developing breast cancer, those receiving extra selenium in their diet had an incidence of breast tumors that was 10 percent lower than those that received no additional selenium. "And there's increasing evidence that many human breast cancers have a similar viral influence," Dr. Schrauzer says. Mice fed a high-fat diet and exposed to cancer-causing chemicals also had fewer, slower-forming tumors with selenium supplementation.

"Human studies with selenium and breast cancer have yet to be done on a large scale," Dr. Schrauzer adds.

To increase your vitamin A intake, look to sweet potatoes, carrots, spinach, cantaloupe, kale, broccoli and winter squash. For vitamin C, drink lots of freshly squeezed orange juice and eat green peppers, papaya, brussels sprouts and more broccoli. Try wheat germ and sunflower seeds for vitamin E. And for selenium, your best bets are seafood, liver and whole grains.

Remember, if you plan to supplement your diet with any of these nutrients, be extremely cautious; large doses of vitamin A (more than 10,000 International Units a day) and selenium (more than 100 micrograms a day) shouldn't be taken without medical guidance.

Eat More Seafood

Besides containing an ample supply of selenium, seafood may prove to be an excellent breast cancer preventive for two reasons. The first has to do with the particular form of polyunsaturated fatty acids found in fish oils; the second has to do with iodine.

Four years of laboratory research conducted while on staff at Memorial Sloan-Kettering Institute for Cancer Research in New York City has led Rashida A. Karmali, M.D., to conclude that fish oil may hold a key to breast cancer prevention.

"My preliminary findings in animal models are still suggestive, not conclusive," she explains. "But evidence is building that marine fatty acids may have a protective effect in the prevention of breast cancer. In the lab, fish oil inhibited the growth of transplanted tumors, blocked development of chemically induced tumors and lowered the level of a putative biomarker—a biochemical indication—of the cancer."

Certainly her theory may help explain epidemiological findings that have long stymied experts: Greenland Eskimos and Icelanders are exceptions to the correlation between high fat intake and high incidence of breast cancer. Dr. Karmali is currently conducting trials on humans to support her laboratory data.

Meanwhile, at the Medical College of Pennsylvania (MCP) in Philadelphia, researchers are continuing their studies on the effects of iodine—another abundant nutrient in seafood—on preventing, diagnosing and treating breast cancer and fibrocystic disease. According to Bernard A. Eskin, M.D., professor of obstetrics and gynecology at MCP, the growth and function of healthy breast cells depend on adequate amounts of iodine. And animal experiments show that when iodine is blocked from breast tissue, breast abnormalities, including cancer, occur and worsen.

Choose Contraception with Care

Whether oral contraceptives contribute to breast cancer is the topic of a continuing debate. In 1983, for example, two studies—both funded by the National Institute of Child Health and Human Development—drew completely different conclusions. One study, which compared Pill use among more than 1,000 women who had different types of cancer with that of 4,000 healthy women, found no correlation between the Pill and breast cancer. Another ten-year study followed 314 patients who developed breast cancer before the age of 37 and found that women under 25 who used high-progestogen oral contraceptivess for five or more years developed cancer at a rate four times the average.

Obviously, the final answers are not yet in. To be on the safe side, ask your doctor to prescribe an oral contraceptive with the lowest dose possible of both estrogen and progestogen. Or better yet, choose another form of birth control. Certainly any woman with a family history of breast cancer should take the more prudent course until we know more.

Express Anger

Some physicians believe that anger suppression—something that was linked with cancer in earlier studies—is still a valid risk factor.

"In the 1950s, two researchers looked at the life history patterns of about 400 cancer patients," Marjorie Brooks, Ph.D., from Jefferson Medical College in Philadelphia, explains. "They found the patients had some very interesting similarities. Many of them seemed unable to express anger or hostility in defense of themselves. The patients could get angry in defense of others or in the defense of a cause. But when it came to self-defense, they didn't follow through.

"Suppressed hostility was another significant factor appearing in some of the other patients. They seemed to lack the discharge mechanism needed to allow anger to surface, so they kept all their anger inside."

Other research, which focused on English women undergoing breast biopsies, "indicated that women who were very, very seldom angry and women who were highly volatile were more likely to have malignant tumors than women who had an appropriate expression of anger," says Dr. Brooks.

Dr. Brooks's own research seems to confirm previous findings. She surveyed 1,100 women who did not have breast cancer and compared the results with those of 15 women with benign tumors and 15 women with malignancies.

"A significantly higher proportion of patients (with both benign and malignant tumors) stated they had experienced much more anger during the previous year than the 1,100 respondents who did not have disease," Dr. Brooks told us. "A larger percentage of women with malignancies had felt angry more often than the women with benign tumors. And a larger percentage of women with benign tumors had felt angrier the previous year than women in normal health."

The *ways* in which the women expressed anger also were different. Women with malignant breast tumors were more likely to apologize for their anger, even when they were right, says Dr. Brooks. So whenever they did express their hostility, they often took it back.

Women with benign tumors tended to get angry and stay angry. Their anger often became an unresolved internal conflict.

Women in normal health were more likely to blow up and then forget about it, says Dr. Brooks. They redirected their attention and energies to more pleasant things.

Keep Calamities in Perspective

Loss of a job, divorce, death of a loved one: traumatic experiences, all of them. And now scientific evidence is underscoring what we've long suspected: Stressful events such as these can suppress the body's immune function, increasing susceptibility to a wide variety of illnesses, including cancer.

Marvin Stein, M.D., and his associates at the Mount Sinai Medical Center in New York City studied the effects of bereavement on the immune function of men whose wives died of breast cancer. Months after their wives died, the men showed a striking decline in white blood cell function, lowering their resistance to infectious disease.

Our response to stressful events may, however, be even more important than the events themselves. At Beth Israel Hospital in Boston, Steven Locke, M.D., director of the psychoneuroimmunology research project there, reports that people who got very upset over stressful events had one-third the level of "natural killer T-cell activity" of people who experienced the same stressful events but were able to deal with them psychologically. (T-cells are a type of white blood cell critical to our immune system.)

In a similar study, Margaret Linn, Ph.D., professor of psychiatry at the University of Miami, found that smokers who developed lung cancer experienced roughly the same traumatic life events as smokers who didn't develop cancer. The difference was that the cancer patients perceived the events to be more stressful and, in some cases, even felt responsible for them.

The moral of these studies is that stressful life events are not worth stewing over. Certainly, a certain amount of grieving following a serious loss or setback is not dangerous and may even be healthy. But if you find yourself in the throes of a depression that you just can't shake, seek professional help. You owe it to your health. (For more on how to cope with stress, see chapter 12.)

C H A P T E R

N I N E

Sexually Transmitted Disease: A Safer Approach to Intimacy

You've read the headlines: an estimated 500,000 persons each year come down with herpes, otherwise known as herpes simplex virus Type I (HSV-I), oral herpes, fever blisters or cold sores. Sometimes accompanied by a fever and swollen gums, the infection is just one of the illnesses that fall under the classification of "sexually transmitted diseases" (STDs). These medical problems, long known as venereal diseases, are now called sexually transmitted diseases partly in an attempt to get away from the long-time stigma of the VD label, which prevented too many people from seeking treatment. (Also, as we explained in chapter 5, certain gynecological infections are sometimes, but not always, transmitted sexually.)

While the risks of certain STDs are potentially very serious—some may cause infertility or even cancer of the cervix if unheeded—most people's fears are exaggerated. Stories that focus on incurability have often alarmed more than informed. While STDs are prevalent, increased awareness of preventive measures, better diagnostic tests, new treatments and the trend to self-help are easing their impact.

Dealing with the Herpes Simplex Virus

Herpes simplex comes in two varieties. Type I usually is associated with distinctive, crusty cold sores on the lips; Type II usually causes painful sores in the genital area.

Herpes of both varieties is easily transmissible. In fact, there is evidence that herpes—particularly the oral variety—is present in the body of most human beings from an early age, says Albert Balows, Ph.D., assistant director for laboratory sciences at the Centers for Disease Control (CDC) in Atlanta.

"They're both related and have a number of characteristics in common. Herpes is unusual in that the virus, particularly Type I, is acquired by almost every human in the early stages of life and doesn't produce any lesions."

Even if herpes is hiding out inside your body, you might live your entire life without a sore. The outward symptoms of herpes can be triggered, however, by stress of almost any type and through fever-producing illness.

"Herpes virus has the unusual ability to hole up in the nerve ganglia. They just get into nerve tissue cells and 'hibernate' there. They can hibernate there a lifetime," according to Dr. Balows.

Personal contact—when and how. Herpes of both varieties is transmitted by personal contact. While most cases of herpes Type I occur on the mouth, lips and nostrils and cases of herpes Type II on the genital organs, we now know that Type II may cause oral outbreaks and Type I may cause sores in the genital area in a small number of cases.

Herpes is transmitted by close body contact—kissing, intercourse, oral or anal sex. The virus lives exclusively in humans.

If you are concerned about catching herpes I or II from someone who has it, it's important to know that the viruses are transmitted only when there are active sores. When the viruses are dormant, says Dr. Balows, it is "virtually impossible" to spread the disease.

Not everyone who is exposed to the viruses will develop symptoms. "For reasons that are not totally understood, some individuals are more susceptible than others," says Dr. Balows.

The dreaded toilet seat. Can you catch herpes from an environmental source? Is it possible to contract genital herpes from a toilet seat in a public restroom, for example? The odds of such a transmission are extremely low.

Trudy Larson, M.D., and Yvonne Bryson, M.D., of the UCLA School of Medicine, conducted a study in which a herpes Type II patient, who had sores on the backs of his thighs, sat on a plastic toilet seat. The study showed that the virus survived for an hour and a half. However, according to Dr. Bryson, "It would be very unlikely you would catch it that way." For one thing, she says, herpes II sores usually are found on and about the genitals and, less frequently, on the buttocks or the thighs. Furthermore, for a second person to contract the virus, the skin on that person's thighs or buttocks probably would have to be broken. "Skin is a good barrier," says Dr. Bryson. "Herpes II doesn't penetrate intact skin."

For the genitals to come into contact with the virus, a person would have to be sitting on the seat in an unusual way.

Dr. Bryson's verdict on toilet-seat transmission of herpes: "It's not a real public health hazard. We have no documented cases of transmission in this fashion."

Contact lens hygiene. It's possible to transmit herpes Type I to the eyes by touching your eyes with your fingers after they've come into contact with a herpes-infected mouth. People who wear contact lenses, for example, are vulnerable, particularly those who wet their lenses with saliva. Herpes in the eye—ocular herpes—can cause blindness. People who wear contact lenses need to be instructed to maintain strict discipline in the removal, cleaning and sterilization of their lenses. "It has to be a procedure that's followed virtually like a religious doctrine," says Dr. Balows.

As for those who persist in wetting their lenses with saliva, he adds, "They're asking for it. They're just red-hot candidates for ocular herpes. It's unusual but it should never exist."

Pregnancy and childbirth. Herpes can be transmitted to a newborn during childbirth. The result is often death.

Viruses from active genital herpes sores in the mother find their way into the baby's bloodstream and ultimately into the brain, causing herpes encephalitis. Doctors can't do much to prevent an outbreak of genital herpes in the mother, but, to reduce the risk, babies born to these mothers frequently are delivered by cesarean section.

Condoms, yes; kissing, no. Is there a way to avoid catching herpes? If your mate is suffering through an outbreak of oral herpes, kissing is, or should be, verboten. As for genital herpes, it's been found in simulated testing that intact condoms provide an effective physical barrier against herpes II. However, many doctors still recommend abstinence when herpes sores are present.

Drug offers relief, not cure. If you have genital herpes, a relatively new drug, acyclovir, has been demonstrated effective in reducing the pain of herpes and shortening the period of the virus's activity. In the long term, progress is being made on a vaccine to prevent herpes in those who have not had the disease, but such a vaccine probably won't help those who already have herpes.

Chlamydia: A New Threat

Another highly contagious infection that has become epidemic is chlamydia (pronounced *kluh-MID-ia*), which is also transmitted during sexual intercourse. This type of STD now occurs between five and ten times as frequently as gonorrhea in women and three times as often in men. Worse, it can often be misdiagnosed.

Chlamydia is caused by an intermediate organism (neither virus nor bacteria) that invades the mucus-producing cells that line the genital tract. The infection is as subtle as it is slow. Typically, the incubation period can last three weeks. Eventually, women will notice a slight discharge, pain during coitus and, later, lower abdominal pain and a fever. In men, the first signs of chlamydia are pain while urinating and a discharge from the urethra.

Don't ignore symptoms. When symptoms appear, it's important to seek medical attention immediately to control the infection.

The organism can pass through the reproductive tract of women, from the cervix to the uterine lining and to the fallopian tubes, if unchecked. There it can prompt pelvic inflammatory disease (PID), scarring the tubes and even resulting in infertility. Male sufferers of chlamydia have similar worries if the disease spreads. The infection can go from the urethra to the testicles, where it can prompt painful swelling and inflammation known as epididymitis, and may result in sterility. Also, more than half of what doctors used to call nonspecific urethritis (NSU), or nongonococcal urethritis (NGU), in men is believed to be caused by the chlamydial organism.

Antibiotics are effective. Once chlamydia is diagnosed, it can be readily treated with antibiotics. Be sure to follow your physician's prescription to the letter, even if your symptoms disappear, since the organism often resists treatment and requires a full course of antibiotics to squelch it.

AIDS

The virus that causes acquired immune deficiency syndrome (AIDS) is far more insidious than the herpes viruses or any one of the viruses that cause colds. The virus in question has a name: human T-cell lymphotropic virus, or HTLV-III. HTLV-III attacks white blood cells called T4 lymphocytes. These cells, derived from the thymus gland, play a key role in our body's defenses against infection and disease.

HTLV-III has a voracious appetite for T-cells. It hijacks the cells, forces them to stop doing what they normally do, and demands that the cells reproduce more viruses like itself.

"When it has utilized its substance within the cell, the lymphocyte shrivels up and the virus escapes and invades other T4 cells," says the CDC's Dr. Balows. As a result of this systematic cell wipeout, the host—the virus's human victim—is deprived of immunity. Consequently, the victim is susceptible to any one of a number of infections that would not normally present a challenge to the immune system.

"Organisms already in the body will take advantage of this to overgrow," says Dr. Balows. "It's like a weed in your yard. Over time it will kill the host."

About 80 percent of those who develop AIDS can be expected to die. There is as yet no cure for AIDS, which afflicts homosexuals, intravenous drug abusers, blood-transfusion recipients and heterosexuals who come into contact with the virus through contact with bisexuals.

There's a related malady called AIDS-related complex (ARC). This simply means that a person carries the virus, but his body is essentially holding its own against the invader. Over time, ARC could progress to a full-blown case of AIDS, remain essentially unchanged or appear to improve, for reasons that are unknown.

This doesn't mean the virus goes away. In fact, it appears to remain dormant in the body.

By the same token, there's a percentage of people who are infected with AIDS but who don't show signs of the disease. "We don't know yet what this means," says Dr. Balows.

Lowering your risks. AIDS is contagious. How do you catch it? Primarily through sexual contact between homosexuals and, to a limited degree, through heterosexual contact with infected bisexual partners. Among intravenous drug abusers, the disease spreads as a result of shared needles. Drug abusers have low resistance to disease in any case.

Those who worry about getting AIDS from a blood transfusion should know that there now is a test administered to blood donors that effectively screens out AIDS-infected individuals. For hemophiliacs, who also were considered at risk, the threat has been substantially minimized by means of a new process in which the clotting factor hemophiliacs need to live is heated, thus killing the AIDS virus.

Dr. Balows says he expects blood-transfusion-transmitted AIDS to decrease "as long as we keep up our guard."

Those more at risk are highly sexually active homosexuals. "That level of promiscuity just increases the risk of exposure," says Dr. Balows. Homosexuals can reduce the risk by a change in lifestyle—fewer sex partners and greater selectivity, perhaps even monogamy.

According to Dr. Balows, there is no evidence at this time that AIDS can be transmitted through fomites (towels, clothing, dishes and other inanimate objects). Many who are likely to come in contact with potential AIDS carriers (doctors, nurses, barbers, ambulance attendants, undertakers and so on) have expressed concern, however.

Should the barber toss away his brush and comb? Should the undertaker take extraordinary care in embalming the corpse of an AIDS victim? Should the paramedic worry about mouth-to-mouth resuscitation?

"All we can tell them is to do as you normally would," recommends Dr. Balows. "You don't have to throw away your comb and brush." As for undertakers, if they follow the usual scientific procedures in embalming the body, there should be no problem.

The AIDS virus has been found to be present in saliva, though there's no evidence that it can be transmitted by kissing, even passionate kissing. But Dr. Balows doesn't recommend it. "It just stands to reason, if you know there's a tiger in the cage, you just don't walk into the cage," he says.

Can you get AIDS from mouth-to-mouth resuscitation? "You can't give out written guarantees that you can't transmit it through mouth-to-mouth, but it's so unlikely as not to create a risk group," says Dr.Balows.

Is a vaccine on the way? Research is progressing, but there have been no definitive results. In any event, a vaccine would be useful in preventing AIDS but probably wouldn't help those already suffering.

Cutting Down on Sexual Risks

Although any intimate contact puts you at risk for sexually transmitted diseases, "women who have multiple sex partners are at highest risk for gynecological infections out of sheer probability from increased exposure," says Mary-Ann Shafer, M.D., associate director of the adolescent medicine unit, department of pediatrics, University of California at San Francisco. The same holds true for men, of course.

Your method of contraception can also have an impact on your susceptibility. Condoms, for instance, are considered the single most important barrier against sexually transmitted diseases *and* gynecological infections. They work in two ways. First, condoms prevent semen, a good culture medium for bacterial growth, from spilling into the vagina. Second, they act as a wall between the penis and the vagina, guarding against the transmission of organisms. The "bugs" they can stop include *Trichomonas, Hemophilus vaginalis* and *Chlamydia.*

Doctors are still debating whether the herpes virus can pass through the pores of a condom under real-life conditions. "No one knows for sure whether condoms protect against herpes," says Dr. Shafer. "But until we know, use a condom between herpes attacks and abstain from intercourse during them."

C H A P T E R

T E N

Birth Control after 35

It's one of those questions that has no easy answer: What kind of birth control is best for an older woman's health?

Is an intrauterine device (IUD) better or worse than the Pill? Is a diaphragm a better method than the IUD? Will the Pill protect me from cancer or put me at risk for cancer? Should I abandon the Pill altogether?

Confused? It's no wonder.

"The contraceptive need of a woman is a very individual thing, and as she gets older—beyond 35—what's best for her may not be what was best for her when she was 25," says Gerald S. Bernstein, M.D., professor of obstetrics and gynecology at the University of Southern California Medical School and director of the family planning clinic at Women's Hospital, Los Angeles.

But the Pill? After 35? "Yes," comes the resounding reply, *if* the woman does not smoke, *if* the woman is in good health and *if* the woman has no personal or family history of heart disease, high blood pressure, hyperlipidemia (elevated triglycerides and cholesterol) or other risk factors.

"She can keep on taking the Pill right up to age 40 if she cares to do so," says Elizabeth Connell, M.D., professor of gynecology and obstetrics at Emory University School of Medicine and a noted authority and researcher on the Pill.

"Misconceptions about the Pill are astounding," says Dr. Connell, "yet the birth control pill has been under more study than any drug in mankind's history.

"You just can't compare the Pill of today to the Pill of 10 or even 5 years ago," she says. "And you certainly can't compare it to the Pill that first came out 25 years ago." The original birth control pill, Enovid 10, contained 150 micrograms of estrogen and 10 milligrams of progestin. Today's pills contain 50 or less micrograms of estrogen and just 1 milligram of progestin.

"As the dosages have come down, down, down, so have many of the risks," comments John J. LaFerla, M.D., associate professor of obstetrics and gynecology at the University of Michigan Medical School and medical director of the Great Lakes Region for the Planned Parenthood Federation of America.

"There has been a lot of scare about the risks involved in taking the Pill after 35," says Dr. Bernstein, "but the risks are not related to age as much as they are related to smoking."

Statistics show that of the ten million U.S. women who take birth control pills, 500 deaths a year are attributed to its use—less than one hundredth of 1 percent. But, the same statistics show that the number could be reduced to 200 if no woman of *any* age who took the Pill smoked—and some 40 percent of birth control pill users do.

But statistics and the doctors we talked to point out that the Pill may prevent more deaths and illnesses than it causes. If the Pill causes 500 deaths a year, it also prevents 850 deaths from ovarian cancer. And of the 9,400 Pill-related hospitalizations each year, six times that many are averted because of the Pill's protective quality.

"The Pill provides protection against ovarian cancer, endometrial cancer, ovarian cysts and pelvic inflammatory disease [PID]," notes Dr. LaFerla.

Nevertheless, it is a fact that the Pill can cause death, and that 90 percent of the 500 deaths a year fall in one category—women 35 and older. And if you eliminate smokers *and* the women in this age group, the yearly death rate would drop to 70 women.

What Are Your Chances?

The table below gives the failure rates for all forms of contraception, divided into two age groups: women under 22 and women 30 and older. (Figures are based on use after one year.) Because a woman's chances of conceiving decline as she ages, the failure rates for older women are lower than for younger women.

Method	Women under 22 (%)	Women 30 and Older (%)
The Pill	4.7	2.1
IUD	9.1	3.9
Condom	20.6	2.2
Spermicides	32.0	15.0
Diaphragm	33.1	15.6
Rhythm	40.8	19.8

SOURCE: Adapted from *Evaluating the Health Risks and Benefits of Birth Control Methods* (New York: The Alan Guttmacher Institute, 1983).

Sterilization Favored

"The reality is, though, that most women past 40 don't take the Pill," says Dr. Bernstein, "and women past the age of 35 are often advised against it by their doctors." In fact, two-thirds of all women 35 and older depend on sterilization to prevent pregnancy, making it, not the Pill, the number one contraceptive choice in the United States.

Astounding? It may be. But it's a fact. Of the 33 million women in the United States practicing contraception, 11.6 million have opted for sterilization either for themselves or for their mates.

Doctors agree that for couples whose families are complete, sterilization is an ideal method. There is no ongoing maintenance, and it is close to 100 percent effective, making it worry free. Either partner can undergo sterilization, and the death rate is very low—about 30 a year, and that's for women only. There have been no reports in the United States of any deaths following vasectomies. "The complications of sterilization are the same as for any surgery," says Dr. Bernstein. "The anesthesia is the major concern. And since a vasectomy is done under a local anesthetic in a doctor's office, this risk is avoided."

Beyond the complications of surgery, side effects of tubal ligation are practically nonexistent. It doesn't disrupt the female reproductive system. A woman still produces hormones, still has a normal menstrual period and still releases eggs. But the chances of fertilizing one of those eggs are pretty slim, which is why the procedure is considered permanent.

"Tubal ligation should not be considered a reversible operation by any woman who opts for it," says Dr. Bernstein, "although the operation is potentially reversible." So a woman should agree to it only if she's sure she doesn't want a baby.

"Some men are scared to death to have a vasectomy," says Dr. Bernstein. "They just have a different perspective of their genitals than women do."

Frederika S. Moxon Heller, M.D., a gynecologist practicing in Berks County, Pennsylvania, says that some men tend to put the burden on the woman. "They figure she's used to being operated on, and if she's had a baby she's used to having a doctor doing things to her body. She is more used to dealing with the medical world. In fairness, it should be something the couple should discuss—should she or he [undergo sterilization]?"

Sterilization may be a fine choice for women who don't want to get pregnant. But what if you want to keep your options open? What do you do if you're over 35 and smoke and can't take the Pill? What if you're over 40 and don't want to take the Pill? What if your general health doesn't allow you to risk the Pill? Then what do you do?

"Use a barrier method," says Dr. Heller. "Or an IUD."

The Risks of IUDs

The IUD, of course, like the Pill, has had its share of bad publicity. While the death rate is low—about 30 per year—its hospitalization rate is even higher than that for the Pill. Some 9,600 women enter hospitals each year due to complications resulting from their IUDs.

Then there's the fact that not every woman can handle an IUD. Some 10 percent of women expel them, and side effects—cramps, breakthrough bleeding, longer and heavier periods—are common, making it an unsatisfactory choice for some. And the wide variety of IUDs that has been on the market over the years has caused a wide range of reactions, from out-and-out furor (caused by the now-off-the-market Dalkon Shield) to wide acceptance (for the copper-containing IUDs that are getting favorable results today).

Still, IUDs are clearly not for everyone.

Weighing the Risks

Of all the reversible methods of birth control available today, only two—the birth control pill and the intrauterine device (IUD)—carry an element of risk that could require hospitalization. Although the risks of complications are low—less than one-tenth of 1 percent for the Pill and four-tenths of 1 percent for the IUD—it's in your own best interest to exercise a little caution and know the symptoms that could spell danger.

IUD

Warning signs:

- Missed period (this could indicate ectopic pregnancy)
- Severe pelvic pain
- Fever

Who should avoid this method:

- Women who have a history of pelvic inflammatory disease
- Women who have multiple partners
- Women who have never had children

"I wouldn't recommend that any woman who doesn't have any children and wants to have children use an IUD," says Dr. Heller. "You're risking pelvic inflammatory disease and risking infertility, and it's just not worth it."

Because of the infection risk, Dr. Heller also says an IUD is not a good choice for women with multiple partners. "For such a woman, a condom might be a better choice."

The other doctors we consulted also spoke highly of the condom, as well as other barrier methods such as the diaphragm, spermicides and the contraceptive sponge.

"I like barrier methods," says Dr. Connell. "If you use them

The Pill

Warning signs:

- Hot, swollen veins, particularly in the back of the leg
- Simultaneous occurrence of shortness of breath, fast heartbeat and severe chest pain

Who should avoid this method:

- Women with a history or family history of thromboembolic disorder (such as phlebitis), stroke, heart disease, benign liver tumor or cancer of the breast or reproductive system
- Women with impaired liver function or acute or chronic liver disease
- Women with high blood pressure
- Women with leg injuries
- Women with gallbladder disease
- Women about to undergo surgery

properly, they can be highly reliable. You must keep in mind, too, that as a woman grows older she gets less and less fertile.

"The diaphragm is a wonderful method, but many women don't like it because it's a hassle," she says. For the same reason, some women don't like spermicides. "They're an interruption. The contraceptive sponge, however, is an excellent method because it doesn't interfere with spontaneity."

The failure rates for *all* forms of contraception are, for the most part, not the fault of the device but the fault of the user. "The caveats are all the same," says Dr. Connell. "Use them correctly."

"There's one important thing that every woman should keep in mind," says Dr. LaFerla. "The risks [from unwanted pregnancy and childbearing] of not using any method of birth control are higher than the risks of any method of birth control, except for older women who smoke."

So if you don't want to get pregnant, don't depend on your luck.

CHAPTER ELEVEN

What You Should Know about Estrogen and Brittle Bones

As a woman, you may be in greater need than men of prevention against osteoporosis, a disease that gradually steals strength-building calcium from bones. All told, an estimated 15 to 20 million Americans suffer from osteoporosis, but the disease is four times more common in women than in men. While women past menopause are the prime victims, the damage begins much earlier in life.

The Risk Factors

To get an idea if you'll be standing tall in years to come or if you'll be one of the millions for whom even a simple task could be back-breaking, see if any of the following risk factors for osteoporosis apply to you.

Advancing age means bone strength retreats. It usually isn't until after age 50 or so that neglected bones start demanding attention—usually by fracturing or shortening your stature. Menopause occurs around this time, taking the biggest toll of all on the

Food Sources of Calcium

Food	Portion	Calcium (mg.)
Sardines, drained	4 oz.	494
Yogurt, skim	1 cup	489
Salmon, drained	4 oz.	365
Milk, skim	1 cup	302
Swiss cheese	1 oz.	272
Monterey Jack cheese	1 oz.	212
Muenster cheese	1 oz.	203
Mozzarella cheese, part skim	1 oz.	183
Dandelion greens, cooked	½ cup	147
Tofu	4 oz.	145
Pizza, cheese	⅛ of 14-in. pie	144
Collards, cooked	½ cup	110
Kale, cooked	½ cup	103
Almonds	¼ cup	83
Chick-peas, dried	¼ cup	75
Cottage cheese, low-fat	½ cup	69
Broccoli, cooked	½ cup	68
Artichoke	1 med.	61
Filberts	¼ cup	60
Eggs	2 large	56

SOURCES: Adapted from *Nutritive Value of American Foods in Common Units,* Agriculture Handbook No. 456, by Catherine F. Adams (Washington, D.C.: Agricultural Research Service, U.S. Department of Agriculture, 1975).

Composition of Foods: Dairy and Egg Products, Agriculture Handbook No. 8-1, by Consumer and Food Economics Institute (Washington, D.C.: Agricultural Research Service, U.S. Department of Agriculture, 1976).

skeletal system. The diet of an older person is often too poor to maintain bone integrity. And with increasing age, the intestines become less efficient at absorbing what calcium there is in the diet. The number of people over age 65 in the United States is expected to reach 22 percent by the year 2050, making osteoporosis one of the medical profession's top research priorities.

While both sexes unavoidably lose some bone mass simply due to aging, most cases of advanced osteoporosis are in women. The fact that women have smaller frames than men may be one explanation for the inequity—when the body needs calcium elsewhere and calls on bones to give up part of their supply, men's bones simply have more in reserve.

Menopause, either natural or surgical, means increased risk. Estrogen, the multitalented hormone produced by a woman's ovaries, helps maintain bone mass and strength in addition to its sex-related duties. When menopause shuts down the supply, bones are more susceptible to fractures. Scientists confirmed this estrogen/bone-strength link when they began seeing premature osteoporosis in premenopausal women who had had their ovaries removed. Hormones may also help account for the female bias in osteoporosis. Testosterone, a male hormone helpful for bone mass, has a more gradual decline in production than estrogen does with its somewhat here-today, gone-tomorrow departure. Women who have spent years taking estrogen-containing birth control pills are thought to enjoy greater protection from osteoporosis, also.

Caucasian and Oriental women are at greater risk than black women. Large-scale studies have repeatedly shown much higher rates of osteoporosis in fairer-skinned races. Two theories may account for this, says Diane Meier, M.D., co-director of the osteoporosis and metabolic bone disease program at Mount Sinai Medical Center, New York City. She's conducting a study of 150 white women and 150 black women, ages 26 to 65, to see if the former have a genetic predisposition to excessive bone loss, or if nutritional habits and body composition are the key. "Blacks, at least in the North American population, tend to have higher obesity rates. And obesity is protective against bone loss," Dr. Meier explains. (Very thin people, then, are also at greater risk.) Black people may have larger, denser bone structures, too, which may give them an advantage against osteoporosis.

A diet short on calcium will mean bone loss in the long run. Scientists found women who had a calcium-rich diet in childhood and early adulthood built a bone mass more able to withstand osteoporosis in later years. Lactose, a carbohydrate in calcium-laden milk, may help the body absorb calcium. Major health organizations are urging people to start getting the U.S. Recommended Daily Allowance of calcium (800 milligrams for children under the age of four, 1,000 milligrams for adults and children four or more years of age and 1,300 milligrams for pregnant and lactating women) early in life, but most Americans barely obtain half these amounts.

Constant dieters lose more than pounds. They risk losing bone mass, too, after years of passing up high-fat (but also high-calcium) dairy products. Low-fat dairy products like skim milk and cottage cheese can help dieters meet their calcium needs.

Strict vegetarians may restrict their bones' strength. "Pure vegetarians who don't eat any dairy products have a hard time getting adequate calcium," says Dr. Meier. "The green vegetables they eat, like broccoli and spinach, do have calcium, but they also contain oxalates, which block the absorption of calcium in the gut."

A meat-eater's diet may eat away at bone strength. A culinary love affair with red meat puts overindulgers at greater risk—studies indicate high protein levels speed up the excretion of calcium in urine and keep the mineral from making its way to bones.

A vitamin D deficiency could mean low-grade bone strength. Vitamin D is normally obtained in adequate amounts through a healthy diet and through the skin with 10 to 20 minutes of sun exposure daily. It's crucial for intestinal absorption of calcium and bone remodeling. But older people may run into a vitamin D shortage due to poor nutrition and long housebound periods due to illness or injury. The sunshine/vitamin D connection is also why people who live in rainier, cloudier climates are thought to be at higher risk than those on whom the sun always shines.

A family history of osteoporosis is related to risk of getting the disease. A woman's grandmother, mother and aunt may provide a clue to what may be in store for her. One theory behind this is that if female relatives reached menopause at a rather early age, they may pass along that tendency, so more years are spent without estrogen's bone protection.

A lazybones lifestyle leads to thinner bones later. One of the many beneficial effects of exercise on the body is the way it helps build bones. Any weight-bearing exercise stimulates the skeleton to put down new bone. Tennis players, weight lifters, ballet dancers and other athletes show wider bones and more cortical, or outside-layer, bone in limbs involved in their particular sport. And astronauts are prime examples of gravity's usefulness—when they're weightless in space, they lose a significant amount of bone mass. Patients confined to bed face a similar situation and can lose as much as 1 percent of their trabecular, or inner, bone per week. Resuming normal weight-bearing activity gradually restores the bone.

Certain substances make calcium seep away. Prolonged use of aluminum-containing antacids, prednisone- or cortisone-containing drugs and diuretics can increase the risk of bone loss. Excessive sodium in the diet is also being explored as a possible cause of calcium excretion, but this research is still very preliminary.

Medical disorders may be additional risk factors for bone loss. Diabetes, hyperthyroidism, hyperparathyroidism, Cushing's disease, rheumatoid arthritis and gastrectomy have been reported to cause osteoporosis, but scientists note the need for more research in this area.

Cigarette smoking may weaken bones. Smoking is suspected of exerting a possibly toxic effect on bone mass. Women who smoke have lower estrogen levels, tend to be thinner and undergo menopause at an earlier age than nonsmokers. Overall, women smokers appear to have lower cortical bone mass.

Alcohol may abuse bones. Heavy alcohol use is one of the few things that puts a man at risk for osteoporosis. Alcoholic men have lower bone mass and lose bone more rapidly than nonalcoholics. In women, the incidence of hip fractures increases as alcohol intake rises. These associations could stem from a direct toxic effect of alcohol, poor nutrition, lower body weight, liver disease or other alcohol-related factors.

The medical profession now offers screening clinics, treatment programs and extensive public education campaigns geared to people at risk. The recommended steps for long-lasting bones are easy for everyone.

Getting adequate calcium and exercise are the best ways to build up healthy bone mass and are important for people of all ages, especially

A Closer Look

There are several ways, some better than others, to tell how bones are holding up *before* they take on the familiar dowager's hump or steal a person's height.

The earliest detection method for bone loss used standard x-rays. But because they were so insensitive, a 20 to 30 percent loss had to occur before the condition was visible.

Radiogrammetry measured changes in thickness of cortical finger bone and was a fairly good way to follow patients, but changes still had to be relatively marked to show up.

"Changes in outer-layer cortical bone are very late reflectors of osteoporosis," explains Gordon DePuey, M.D., director of the division of nuclear medicine at Emory University Hospital and member of the department of radiology, nuclear medicine division, at Emory University School of Medicine, Atlanta. "The spongy, inner trabecular bone is what you need to see if you want to be accurate. This is what primarily composes vertebrae."

One method still used today is single-photon absorptiometry, which measures a portion of the wrist. "This is accurate enough to detect slight changes in bone," says Dr. DePuey, "but it still measures primarily cocortical bone. People who checked out okay at the wrist were winding up with hip and vertebral fractures later."

those under age 35. Adequate calcium from dairy products, green vegetables, sardines and salmon with edible bones, tofu and other food sources or from dietary supplements is essential. Weight-bearing exercise should be done at least five times a week, and it can be anything from walking to tennis.

Be sure to get some sunshine and maintain adequate vitamin D in your diet. Finally, minimize the risk factors in your control, like smoking and alcohol.

One step up is dual-photon absorptiometry, the most popular method today. This can measure bones deeper in the body, like the hip and lumbar vertebrae, and can detect even a 4 percent change. Both single and dual absorptiometry take only a short while and use just one-third the radiation of a chest x-ray.

"There's no risk from this low level of radiation," notes Dr. DePuey, "and the machines are springing up at centers everywhere because they're very affordable. The tests are covered by most insurance companies, too."

Computerized tomography is another very accurate method of measuring bone mineral density, but it is less frequently used due to somewhat higher cost and greater radiation exposure.

A conceptual breakthrough was made at the National Aeronautics and Space Administration's Ames Research Center, where a device measures the strength of astronauts' skeletons and determines if there are risk factors associated with weightless space flight. Donald Young, Ph.D., a physiologist in the biomedical research division, came up with the idea for the Bone Stiffness Analyzer, the fastest, most accurate and unique measuring device yet. It uses no radiation, just vibrations bounced off bone and recorded by a sensor. Researchers at Stanford Medical Center are testing the device as a prelude to commercial development.

Starting the Treatment

With one possible exception, nothing seems to replace bone once it's lost after menopause. Fluoride looks promising for rebuilding bone, but it has not yet been approved by the U.S. Food and Drug Administration (FDA) for mass use.

"Women approaching menopause need to consult with their physicians for assessment or diagnosis and should ask about treatment and prevention of the disorder," notes Sandra Raymond, executive director of the National Osteoporosis Foundation in Washington, D.C.

After taking your history and assessing your risk for the disease, doctors at screening clinics can examine the condition of your bones with quick and accurate procedures. (See the accompanying box.) If bone seems to be ebbing or your history makes you a likely candidate, you can begin treatment to keep the condition from getting worse.

A boost in calcium is urged by most researchers, even though calcium's postmenopausal role hasn't been documented as well as its effectiveness in building strong bone in childhood and through early adulthood. Doctors suggest 1,000 to 1,500 milligrams of calcium for women at menopause and beyond. This is also about the same amount taken by astronauts after missions.

"If you're taking a supplement," advises Dr. Meier, "take it with juice or fluid independently of meals. Try it first thing in the morning, an hour before breakfast. The juice will stimulate gastric acid for absorption, and the delay of breakfast will ensure protein and fiber won't compete with calcium in the gut for absorption."

Walking wins out as the most recommended exercise for postmenopausal women, again done at least five times a week. But the biggest gun in the fight against further bone loss is estrogen supplementation.

The FDA has just approved low-dose estrogen to retard further bone loss in postmenopausal women with evidence of loss or deficiency of bone mass. The labeling also states that the estrogen should be used with other measures, such as calcium and exercise. Provided that a woman's health poses no contraindications to estrogen, the therapy seems to be as safe as it is effective.

One study of over 500 women found estrogen users had significantly greater mineral content, fewer wrist and hip fractures and greater cortical thickness than women who didn't receive estrogen. "Long-term estrogen-replacement therapy confers significant protection against bone loss and fracture," the researchers note.

Women with either a personal or family history of endometrial or breast cancer probably should not have estrogen therapy, cautions Dr. Meier. "There's a marked increase in endometrial cancer in people taking postmenopausal estrogen replacements. But endometrial cancer is very treatable and less risky than a hip fracture, which has a very high mortality rate."

If doctors find severe bone loss has already taken place and estrogen doesn't seem feasible, fluoride in combination with calcium might be used to try to reverse the damage. Generally this treatment is not used as the first line of defense against osteoporosis.

Stress-Coping Skills for Mind and Body

Traditionally, stress has been considered a male malady. But women are catching up in this arena, even though they may lag behind in others.

Ever since the 1960s, women have vied with men for positions in politics, the workplace, science, sports and even outer space. But the latest news is that women are now competing with men for rising rates of alcoholism, lung cancer, ulcers and heart disease.

What the current news stories aren't saying, however, is that women can reverse this trend.

The Stress of Being a Woman

The first step in stress control is to recognize that the *causes* of stress differ for men and women.

Abrupt change. Georgia Witkin-Lanoil, Ph.D., a member of the clinical faculty in the psychiatry department of Mount Sinai Medical College and author of *The Female Stress Syndrome,* says that abrupt change is one of the culprits causing women's stress.

Dr. Witkin-Lanoil explains that in 1967, researchers Thomas

Holmes and Richard Rahe developed the now-famous Social Readjustment Rating Scale, a means of rating a number of life's events and the stress these events cause. According to this scale, the more life changes a person experiences in a given year, the more prone she is to stress and related illnesses. "The people who have been undergoing the most change recently or who are most directly affected by life's events—from divorce to pregnancy to alterations in home responsibility—are women."

Today, women of all ages are experiencing changes in roles. There are the teenager and the single woman who face new relationships, the homemaker who works without peer support, the working mother who juggles a career and family life, and the woman who is getting older in a youth-oriented society. These changes often mean fewer role models, fewer support systems and more stress.

Helen DeRosis, M.D., associate clinical professor of psychiatry at New York University Medical Center and author of *Women and Anxiety*, believes that with changing roles and new challenges comes anxiety or fear of the unknown. And too much anxiety can lead to too much stress.

Lack of control. Changing roles are only half of the story. "How much control women feel they have in a situation plays a large part in stress, especially when it comes to work-related situations," says Paul Rosch, M.D., clinical professor of medicine at New York Medical College and president of the American Institute of Stress. He explains that although recent studies have shown that work-related stress is the number one health problem, it is *not* the female execs and bosses who are getting the angina or ulcers. "It's those who are bossed and who have relatively little control over their own decisions." And the people who are in those kinds of jobs are predominantly women.

Great expectations; low wages. What can lead to even more stress, says Dr. Rosch, is that although expectations for female workers are higher, wages are lower. Also, women often face discrimination and sexual harassment on the job. What's more, women receive relatively little support from society or at home in the form of child care or flexible time schedules. Despite women's changing roles, says Dr. Rosch, the prevailing attitude is that a woman is still expected to "act like a lady, think like a man and work like a dog." No wonder women are driven to drink at alarming rates!

Dr. Witkin-Lanoil agrees that stress is not just a result of women's changing roles. "Female stress is more a result of dual roles," she says. Women not only move into new roles but also retain the old roles. The woman who works still has to clean the house and care for the kids.

Many women suffer from the superwoman complex and compound their stress themselves, says Dr. Witkin-Lanoil. They believe they must perform *all* their roles perfectly. They also have not learned how to say no to others or how to allow themselves to enjoy a new role without feeling guilty.

Stress in Double Doses

No matter what causes it, the results of chronic stress in women are never good. The whole purpose of stress is to produce chemical, psychological and physiological changes to help us cope with threatening

A Checklist of Stress Signals

Paul Rosch, M.D., of New York Medical College, says there is an increasing tendency for women to develop Type A behavior patterns, which could lead to stress-related illness like heart disease. Take this test and see if your behavior may be steering you toward excess stress. (Check off any of the following statements that apply to you.)

- I work best under a deadline.
- I talk louder and faster than others and emphasize my point by facial expressions or gestures.
- Winning is everything to me, even when playing with children.
- I rarely take time out to "smell the roses."
- I feel that if I want something done, I must do it myself.
- It's not pleasurable for me to lie on a beach and do nothing for a week.

life situations. But when we cannot use a "fight or flight" response, our stress has no outlet. Over time, it collects in our bodies. It's that chronic stress that can aggravate preexisting conditions or bring on new ones like colitis, high blood pressure, asthma, allergies and skin disorders.

Women get a double dose of stress, says Dr. Witkin-Lanoil. In addition to the disorders mentioned, which are common to both sexes, women have certain built-in biological stresses, like menstruation, pregnancy and menopause, that put a tremendous strain on their bodies throughout their life. The combination of these physical stresses with the everyday stresses of life and the special female social stresses adds up to the "female stress syndrome."

That newly named syndrome may include premenstrual symptoms, amenorrhea (absence of menstruation), frigidity, infertility and other serious disorders like anxiety attacks, neurosis, the eating disor-

- I'm impatient when standing in line or following a slow driver.
- I am more concerned with what others think of me than with my own opinion of myself.
- I always feel rushed and usually try to do more than one thing at once.
- I tend to interrupt people.
- I dislike arriving early and waiting around.
- I'd rather do many things fairly well than a few things excellently.

If you feel that nine or more of these statements describe you, you tend to fit the Type A mold, says Dr. Rosch. Perhaps it's time to take a new look at the stress in your life and seek ways to relieve it.

ders anorexia and bulimia, and depressive psychosis. Factors such as individual differences, age, hormone levels and physical fitness can interact to produce the female stress syndrome.

Rx for stress. Stress does not have to be the bottom line to women's changing roles, however. "Women need to give themselves permission to relax," says Dr. Witkin-Lanoil. And the sooner the better. "Don't wait until you are on the verge of a breakdown to acknowledge stress." If you can't give yourself permission to relax, she suggests you find a counselor who will give it to you. She further suggests that women stop feeling guilty and worry less about what they "should" be doing.

Stress Busters

Stress, unfortunately, is here to stay. The trick is to learn to live with stress today to minimize its effects tomorrow.

We're not talking about elaborate exercise programs or expensive escapes to some South Seas island, though. We know you're busy and need effective stopgap solutions to help you deal with stress right now—when you are toe-to-toe with the tensions of everyday life. That's why we've put together 20 quick and easy stress releasers that you can use to diffuse stress and keep you from buckling under in the crunch.

Find which tranquility techniques work for you. Keep this list handy and pull it out whenever you need to put stressful events into proper perspective.

1. Take a hike. When pressures mount to the boiling point, don't just sit there and stew; get up and take a walk. According to Herbert deVries, Ph.D., director of the physiology and exercise laboratory at the University of Southern California, a brisk 10- to 15-minute walk is a good safety valve that has been shown to relieve muscular and nervous tension.

2. Plant a petunia. Digging in the dirt, pruning the hedges or raking the leaves can be therapeutic, breaking down any frustrations you may be feeling, say experts. And puttering around your plants just may have positive benefits for your body, too. "Anytime you garden, there is a release of nervous tension and rechanneling of anxiety," reports Richard Mattson, Ph.D., a horticultural therapist at Kansas State University.

3. Have a "cuppa" tea. Herb tea, that is. Says California herbalist Nan Koehler: "Even the ritual of preparing tea—holding the warm cup in your hands and feeling the steam—can be tremendously soothing and relaxing." Camomile is the most common calming tea. Other herbs noted for their soothing properties include basil, catnip, hops and valerian.

4. Let it all out. Bottled-up anger can boost your blood pressure, give you headaches and possibly lead to ulcers. A healthier response to stress is to calmly confront conflicts head-on. Discuss problems in a detached manner. Go ahead and groan once in a while, too. Some experts believe a good groan vibrates the body, relaxes the muscles and sort of "massages you from the inside out." Another effective pressure valve is to have a good cry. Tears may help relieve stress by ridding the body of potentially harmful chemicals produced in stressful times. Or you might just want to laugh at life a little—or a lot. Laughter diffuses tension and restores perspective.

5. Breathe easy. Your breathing becomes rapid and shallow when you're overwrought. Slow it down and you discharge stress. Try filling your lungs slowly in seven seconds, then take eight seconds to exhale. Train yourself to deep breathe like that to certain triggers—a red light and a ringing telephone are two good ones.

6. Do a slow stretch. Make your muscles relax by gently and slowly stretching a specific set of muscles and visualizing yourself relaxing until you feel a tug. Hold for 10 to 30 seconds and release. This is a good tension releaser to try when you're stuck in traffic: Grasp the top of the steering wheel with both hands, making sure your forearms are also resting on the wheel. Place your buttocks and lower back against the back of the seat. Now hunch your upper body forward, and arch your back like a frightened cat.

7. Shut out "shoulds." Trying to live up to certain imposed images and standards can add to your stress load. Be aware of the stereotypes surrounding you and the pressure to conform—the perfect parent, or the superwoman with the pencil-thin figure. Think of your real self, not your ideal self. Try not to be perfect. Think: "This is who I am, not who I *should* be."

8. Get a little help from your friends. Peer support systems—both inside and outside of home and work—can keep you sane through stressful situations and help you find solutions to problems. They will also keep you healthy. Research indicates that social ties can lower your risk of heart disease, cancer, digestive disorders and even accidents.

9. Give yourself good PR. Progressive Relaxation—tensing muscles and then slowly releasing them—is a good way to banish stress from your body. First, lie down and close your eyes. Make a tight fist, then tense the muscles in your wrist and forearm. Hold for five seconds, feeling the tension, then unclench and let the tension drain from your forearm, wrist and fingers. Note the difference between the feeling of tautness and the pleasure of total relaxation. Now repeat this tension/relaxation sequence for your left hand, then for your upper arms, shoulders, neck, face, legs, feet and toes. Soon you'll be able to perform it anytime and anywhere you find yourself in a stressful situation.

10. Go out and play. "Doing something that's fun and makes you feel joyful can help yank you off the treadmill of your perpetual battle with stress," says Matt Weinstein, Ph.D. Whether it's movies, books, painting or spectator sports, it matters less what you do or for how long you play than that you do it regularly. And if you just can't get away, then play hooky, advises one job-stress expert. A mental-health day, away from everyday tensions, may be just the stress break you may need to renew your energy.

11. Massage your muscles. A gentle foot rub can make you feel good and relaxed all over. Start by applying pressure with your thumbs to your soles, then massage every square inch. Work your toes, too—move them from side to side, forward and back.

12. Take to the tub. A warm or neutral bath dilates the blood vessels, increases circulation to the extremities, relaxes muscles and induces sleep. A cool bath stimulates nerves and acts like a tonic. Both baths are good stress beaters. Try tossing in a few herbs—like lavender—for extra soothing. Or add some sage, salt, seaweed or apple-cider vinegar to take the tension out of weary muscles.

13. Make a daily "to do" list. If you want to reduce stress, one key is to gain control of your time. And that takes planning every day. Simply jot down everything you want to accomplish and then prioritize each time. "A" tasks are those you must do, "B" tasks get done if you have time and "C" tasks are those that are no big deal if they don't get done. You'll probably be surprised to discover that the majority of your tasks are insignificant to your life's goals. "Time management liberates you," says Dennis Jaffe, Ph.D. "It's a way to control pressure and manage the environment." And while you are scheduling, be sure to leave yourself a bit of unstructured time, just to do nothing but experience life as it happens.

14. Head for the hills. Or the ocean, open fields or desert. "Being in a natural surrounding is good for relieving stress," says Aaron Katcher, M.D., an associate professor of psychiatry at the University of Pennsylvania. "Watching the surf or the clouds roll by is a form of meditation. Our thoughts are focused on the rhythm of things, and they're not occupied with problems or worries." Some experts say that a drive to the country or a stroll in the park is as effective as tranquilizers or biofeedback.

15. Repeat a relaxing word. Studies show that saying the same word over and over—preferably one ending in an "m" or "n" sound, such as *calm* or *home*—can help quiet the central nervous system, slow the heart rate and lower the blood pressure.

16. Talk to the animals. Your dog may be more than just your best friend. In fact, he may be your best medicine, too. According to pet therapists, our pets can relax us, help us communicate with each other, build our self-esteem and comfort us when we're down. They may even help us to live longer and reduce our risk of stress-related illnesses like heart disease. Allergic to animals? Don't despair. Some doctors say that just gazing at fish in a tank can be as relaxing as meditation or biofeedback and may lower your blood pressure temporarily.

17. Share the load. Women get stress in double doses because they often take on new roles while holding on to the old roles.

Get your partner to pitch in and divide up the chores. Let your children handle all the responsibility they can. Hire all the help you can afford. Learn to say no to others and yes to yourself. Enjoy your new roles without feeling guilty about your old ones.

18. Use your imagination. Physiologist Mary Asterita, Ph.D., of the Indiana University School of Medicine, reminds us that it's not the events that cause us stress but our negative thoughts about them. Why not play out positive images in your mind and make your imagination work *for* you? Do this by visualizing a tense situation. Imagine that you are trying to walk with an impossibly heavy backpack. Then visualize someone coming along to lighten your load. Imagine the sensations and the relief of the problem-solving process. You might want to think of this as a film you can rewind and play whenever you are facing stressful situations. Another suggestion is to imagine an object, say a rose. Visualize its texture, color and smell. Lose yourself in the sensations of the rose. That kind of focusing is another instant-unwinding technique you can play back in your mind whenever you face tense times.

19. "B" careful. It's easy to neglect your diet during stressful times and to become deficient in certain nutrients, like thiamine and niacin. These B vitamins play crucial roles in mental health—they keep the nervous system functioning. But subsisting on fast food full of refined carbohydrates and sugar-laden soft drinks can use up thiamine reserves. So take a B break whenever you can—reach for seeds, nuts, beans and whole wheat muffins. Or sprinkle some brewer's yeast on your cereal. Steer clear of the B robbers like alcohol, coffee and cigarettes.

20. Think of change as challenge. There is evidence that those who cope most positively with stress consider it natural for things to change. They anticipate changes as a useful stimulus to development. Consequently, they suffer less from the psychological signs of stress like anxiety and depression. So be prepared to cope with stressful situations before they cause strain. If you are involved in a frustrating work situation you cannot change, for example, why not take on the challenge of learning to ski? It just may become a symbol of the possibilities for positive change in your life.